HEALTHY EATING 2 IN 1 VALUE COLLECTION: KICKING THE DIET MINDSET + MOVE ON FROM SUGAR ADDICTION

ULTIMATE GUIDES FOR SUGAR DETOX AND INTUITIVE EATING TO START A SUGAR CLEANSE, STOP BINGE EATING AND EAT CLEAN

GABRIELLE TOWNSEND

SILK PUBLISHING

CONTENTS

KICKING THE DIET MINDSET

Foreword	3
Introduction	7
1. What Is Intuitive Eating?	15
2. Identifying The Problem	30
3. Hunger Is The Enemy	48
4. It's All In Your Head!	56
5. Exercise - The Way to Look and Feel Better	63
6. How Do I Actually Eat Intuitively?	78
7. My 5 Step Process To Success	87
8. Stop Blaming Yourself	93
9. Surround Yourself With the Right Environment	109
10. Seeking Help and Finding a Community	117
Afterword	123
References	131

MOVE ON FROM SUGAR ADDICTION WITH THE SUGAR DETOX CLEANSE

Introduction	141
1. The Emotional Aspects of Sugar Addiction	147
2. Sugar Detox Cleanse Step 1	163
3. Step 2	176
4. Step 3	191
5. Step 4 - Week 1	215
6. Step 5	249
7. The Detox is Done. Now What?	258
Afterword	263
References	265

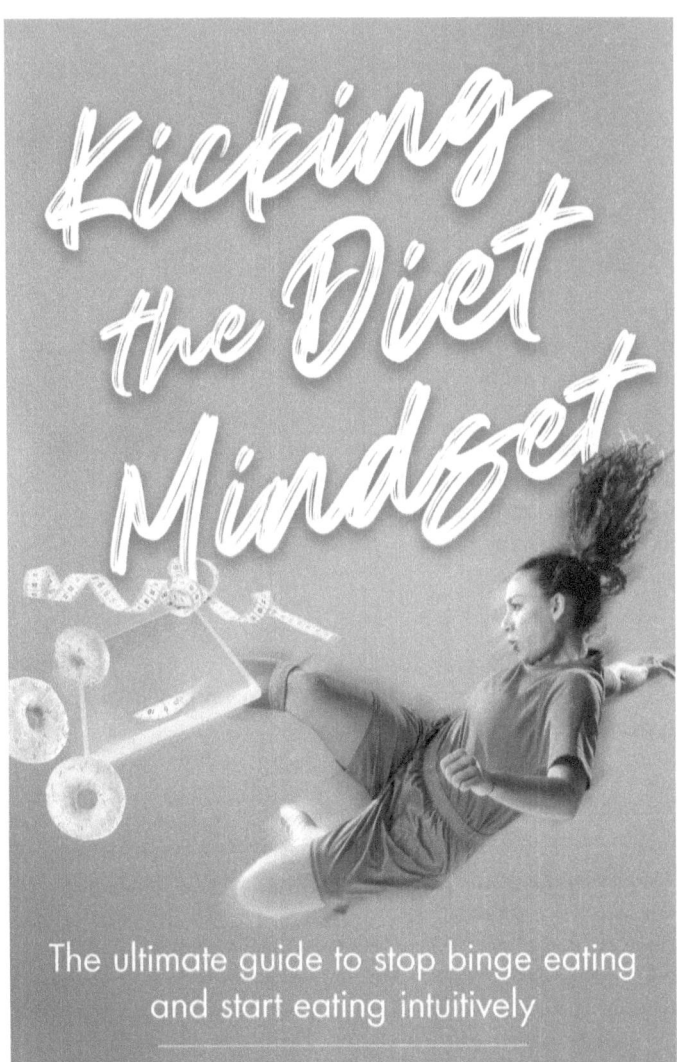

Kicking the Diet Mindset

The ultimate guide to stop binge eating and start eating intuitively

GABRIELLE TOWNSEND

Gabrielle Townsend

© **Copyright 2020 - All rights reserved.**

The content contained within this book may not be reproduced, duplicated or transmitted without direct written permission from the author or the publisher.

Under no circumstances will any blame or legal responsibility be held against the publisher, or author, for any damages, reparation, or monetary loss due to the information contained within this book, either directly or indirectly.

Legal Notice:

This book is copyright protected. It is only for personal use. You cannot amend, distribute, sell, use, quote or paraphrase any part, or the content within this book, without the consent of the author or publisher.

Disclaimer Notice:

Please note the information contained within this document is for educational and entertainment purposes only. All effort has been executed to present accurate, up to date, reliable, complete information. No warranties of any kind are declared or implied. Readers acknowledge that the author is not engaged in the rendering of legal, financial, medical or professional advice. The content within this book has been derived from various sources. Please consult a licensed professional before attempting any techniques outlined in this book.

By reading this document, the reader agrees that under no circumstances is the author responsible for any losses, direct or indirect, that are incurred as a result of the use of the information contained within this document, including, but not limited to, errors, omissions, or inaccuracies.

FOREWORD

If you have a history of constantly being drawn to a new diet or gimmick to help you lose those unwanted pounds and you seem to be getting nowhere slowly, and you've come to the point where you simply don't know who to trust anymore because there are too many conflicting dieting concepts out there—this book is especially for you.

Here you will learn how to take a complete break from what you've been brainwashed into believing: that to be loved by someone, or accepted by society, you need to fit into this size, you need to be this shape, or you need to belong to a community of dieters.

If you're feeling overwhelmed and confused by all the conflicting messages and diets available out there, you've found a solution. Your confusion is natural because there are so many conflicting messages and diets out there. Virtually everywhere you look there's some new miracle cure popping up on your Facebook feed. It's no wonder that the diet industry is thriving: it's a multi-billion-dollar industry after all.

By now, you're probably tired of asking yourself which of the diets out there is right for your age, shape, height, personal preference, blood type, and even your culture? After all, you've probably tried a few and failed more often than not. Many of the diets available start off promising and then all of a sudden you notice the pounds creeping back on, plus a little extra for good measure.

I'm here to burst the dieting bubble and to let you know that none of them are doing you any good at all! Yep, you heard me—the best diet you can be on right now is NO DIET! And no, I'm not the first person to come up with this theory. As a matter of fact, this belief has been kicking around since the 1970s, with it finally being given the official label of "intuitive eating" for the first time in 1995.

What makes this different from every other diet out there? While it's a relatively simple concept, many find it more difficult to learn and apply to their lives daily. Intuitive eating is based on the simple philosophy of eating when you are hungry and stopping when your body is feeling satisfied. It's moving away from starving yourself for extended periods between meals like you would do for example during intermittent fasting.

Another main objective of intuitive eating is to build an effective barrier against binge eating. Intuitive eating is actually the complete opposite of a diet. There's no calorie counting or restriction involved. Because it's designed this way you won't suffer from craving all the goodies on the 'bad food list.' As a matter of fact, there is no good or bad food list with intuitive eating.

FOREWORD

Intuitive eating takes time to learn and practice. It means learning to listen to what your body is telling you, rather than allowing your mind to be in control. Intuitive eating encourages you to eat anything that you want and learning to accept your body image. Learning to love who you are and what you look like. This acceptance is the key to living a life that's happier and more fulfilled, irrespective of what you look like.

In the pages that follow we'll discuss ways to introduce intuitive eating into your life so you can regain control over your lifestyle and never have to diet again.

It will teach you that you can still enjoy the foods you want to eat in moderation without feeling guilty about what you're putting into your mouth. It replaces the constant fear of not being able to fit into your favorite pair of jeans with the freedom to love yourself for who you are, as you are!

INTRODUCTION

"Diets, like clothes, should be tailored to you."

— JOAN RIVERS

Do you suffer from mood swings resulting in feelings of guilt, depression and anxiety constantly because of your addiction to a fad, weight loss gimmick, or diet? Are you one of those shoppers who counts calories on every item before adding it to your cart? This is often happening on a subconscious level and because you've been doing it for so many years, you don't even realize that you're doing it anymore.

Do you feel extreme anxiety and remorse when you've enjoyed a night out with your friends or that special someone, knowing that you've overindulged? Are these sorrowful sentiments likely to linger with you longer than you'd like them to? Or do you try and figure out what your next step is going to be to get rid of the additional calories you've carelessly overindulged in? Are your eating decisions putting you on a "permanent guilt trip" rather than allowing you to enjoy the important things you want and deserve from life?

If you had to identify the category that you fall within, would you admit to being addicted to a diet? There are so many individuals simply going through the motions of life—one with little to no joy because they constantly feel desperately unhappy about what they look like. They don't like the way their clothes fit, and they are permanently uncomfortable about their weight. For these individuals, picking up 500g is too much to deal with, let alone packing on a couple of extra pounds for no reason.

Do you shudder every time you need to visit a medical professional for a routine check-up and they ask you to climb on a weight scale? You're almost waiting for it to show an 'error' reading because it can't handle your weight!

Does the very thought of holidays or special celebrations leave you feeling depressed because you know that it's going to result in any weight you've managed to lose piling right back on again? Is your anxiety worsened by all the traditional 'food-based' holidays like Thanksgiving, Easter, Christmas, Mother's Day, Father's Day, weddings and anniversaries, not to mention any birthdays in between?

Is walking past your local bakery simply too tempting to pass up the chance for fresh bagels or croissants? Can you tie some of your physical anxiety to food? Do you turn to food whenever you're bored or emotional? Or has that extra helping of whatever you ate at dinner left you feeling bloated, uncomfortable and unable to sleep?

If you can relate to any of the above emotions or expe-

INTRODUCTION

riences, this book may just be what you need to regain some of the control over your life. While you may not realize it at this moment, you actually have more control and say in your association with food than you are willing to admit to.

We'd all like to be thin... I mean, who can blame you for feeling this way when everywhere you look, 90 lbs. models adorn glossy magazines, movies, advertisements, and even Instagram. Every woman wants to be the "perfect" size with ideal measurements to match, but let's get real for a moment: we are all unique and different. These differences should be accepted and celebrated rather than send you on a lifelong guilt-trip due to the body type you were born with.

Because of this ideology that's placed on girls from a young age, many women begin dieting from the time they're a teenager and things kind of literally go "pear-shape" from there on out. Yo-yo dieting becomes the norm, each time resulting in more and more weight returning than before. For some, the perfect body only begins to disappear once children arrive! After the first child, things usually get back to normal fairly quickly. By baby number 2 it can become a bit harder. The weight is harder to get off and keep off, especially that bulge directly around the midriff that closely resembles a flotation device. No amount of dieting seems to make even the slightest dent in getting rid of this excess weight that you're constantly carrying around with you wherever you go.

Between the sleepless nights tending to a newborn baby and possibly chasing after another toddler, you'd think that all the excess weight would just melt away

INTRODUCTION

magically. Unfortunately, if you happened to undergo a cesarean section, your chances of getting rid of that spare weight around your waistline make finding a unicorn in your garden to be a more realistic possibility.

Because you're exhausted and emotional, you turn to your comfort food of choice, whatever this may be (and chances are, it's nothing healthy like carrot sticks or a fruit smoothie). It probably resembles something with loads of calories, that you absolutely know you're going to regret in the morning, or whenever you next step on the scale.

Finding the time for an exercise regime is virtually impossible, especially if you need to catch up on your own nap time by synchronizing it with baby for the first few weeks and months.

No matter how old you are, once the dieting merry-go-round begins, it's more and more difficult to get off the longer you remain on it. While diets themselves are restrictive in terms of what you can or can't eat, the effects on your mental health begin to take their toll. Every time you happen to crave that special treat and give in to temptation and indulge, you feel guilty about it and this leads to anxiety, which could, in turn, lead to depression.

In an article written by (Sauer, 2018), she admitted… "I feel anxious about my body and anxious about what I eat. I often find myself overeating when presented with "off-limits" foods and feeling guilty about it far too often."

There's no miracle cure and "one-size-fits-all" when it comes to dieting—why? Because each of us is totally different and unique. We each have different DNA and blood types, our body types are different and for some,

INTRODUCTION

metabolism comes into play. The thyroid can wreak havoc on the entire system making weight loss an impossibility—yet we all still desire the perfect body to make us feel good about ourselves. We feel as though if we have the perfect body all will be right in the world.

Intuitive eating gives us the formula and means to develop another way of life. It deals with not only your physical side but your mental and emotional side as well. It's about learning to listen to your body when making decisions about what you plan on putting into it in terms of what you eat. Listening to your body initially can be tricky and you're bound to have a number of bumps in the road as you begin this exciting new journey off the dieting-merry-go-round!

The main thing with intuitive eating is to trash your thoughts of ever dieting again. It's getting rid of all your previously attempted diets that simply made you more frustrated daily. It's kicking out the Keto recipes, archiving your ancient Atkins diet book, banishing the "Blood Type" diet and any other failed fad your body has never quite responded to. From taking pills that are supposed to magically dissolve fatty deposits around your body to intermittent fasting routines, many of you would have possibly tried a number of these only to have all the weight creep back the moment you stopped.

For those with underlying health issues such as diabetes, heart, lung or back problems that prevent them from participating in the high-intensity exercise programs needed to support each of these diets, there's simply no hope or light at the end of the tunnel. All that this results in is leaving you feeling miserable and dejected.

INTRODUCTION

Personally, I have struggled with the mentality of diets, often losing weight only to gain it all back again, or going all out and destroying any momentum I may have gained by rigidly sticking with the diet by binge eating. I'm the first to admit that dieting for me simply doesn't work and I had to find a new approach to discovering how to eat what I want when I want while being mindful of not only my health but my body as well.

The natural benefit to approaching intuitive eating is discovering joy in your life, rather than constantly being on edge, counting carbs or calories, or cringing every time you walk past a store that sells food that's on your "do not touch" list.

It's actually being able to keep the weight off, instead of an endless yo-yo weight on, weight off effect. It's being confident and comfortable getting on your bathroom scale without worrying about what the numbers say!

Intuitive eating allows me to enjoy those foods that I want when I want them by learning to listen to what my body is telling me.

My main reason for writing *Kicking the Diet Mindset* is that I realized I am the best person—the only person—who can actually make these choices for me. I realized that following every new crazy diet was not the solution that I was looking for, or what was best for me in the long run. I also wanted to share what I have learned about this completely new way of looking at your personal relationship with food with others who may, like I was, totally frustrated with being bombarded constantly with this diet, shake or pill!

With my help and expertise, by following the tips and suggestions in *Kicking the Diet Mindset*, you will be fully equipped to discover and deal with your body image. Whether you are happy with your body right now or not, it's important to get there properly with all the facts at your disposal.

Are you currently keen on trying out yet another diet? Go ahead, but let's look at your history to date, as well as the history of others. If you genuinely want to remain healthy, physically and mentally throughout life it's going to come from knowing yourself and your limits and learning to eat intuitively.

No human is meant to be dieting for 80-plus years: whether healthy or not, it's been proven that people only have a certain capacity for deprivation before they break.

What if you never have to break? What if eating good food and splurging sometimes can actually be fun?

Don't waste another year of your life binge eating and then punishing yourself mentally and emotionally for it.

Every chapter in this book is structured in a way that will provide you with actionable steps that can help you choose what is truly best for your body in both the short and long term. Stop being distracted by every new trend, tool, course or diet (all this is achieving is presenting you with "Shiny Object Syndrome"). Identify what the problem is and fix it immediately.

If you follow the methods outlined in this book, it is very likely that you will never struggle with clarity around dieting again.

1

WHAT IS INTUITIVE EATING?

"As you go through your day, try to look at food differently. Look at how it works for your body: nourishing it, fueling, and allowing pleasure. Notice how food feels friendly when you eat intuitively, if food is there for you as a friend. Can you feel the difference?

— *FOOD: FRIEND AND FUEL? – STAY ATTUNED*

INTRODUCTION TO WHAT INTUITIVE EATING IS

Understanding what intuitive eating is takes us back to how we behaved as children. It's a way of eating that we've forgotten as we moved into adulthood. Instead of drinking a bottle until we were full or eating what was on our plate until we were full, then returning to play, we've become like robots in our eating habits.

Rather than stopping, we eat until the plate is empty,

no matter how big it is, and too often we've piled way too much on the plate in the first place. Intuitive eating promotes a healthy outlook towards the food that we eat and prevent us from over-indulging. The theory behind it is to eat when you are hungry, rather than when you're absolutely ravenous, and to stop eating when you are feeling content or comfortable, rather than bloated due to overeating.

Its name indicates that you should follow your own "intuition" regarding your need for food and feeling satisfied. While this is implied, there are not many individuals who know where this invisible line begins or ends. Imagine that you could measure your hunger on a scale or measuring stick, where zero is the point where you are absolutely starving/ravenous for your next morsel of food, and 10 is the point where you are about to explode because you're feeling totally stuffed (and you know you're going to regret it in the morning)! The scale has different points that measure variations of hunger or being satisfied.

The idea behind intuitive eating is to eat when you are hungry and stop when you are content, or comfortable. Realistically, it's probably ranging between 2 and 7 or 8 on the scale depending on your current size and body type (and yes, your body type can affect all of this). It could also be influenced by other medical factors which we'll cover a bit further on.

Many people don't know how to measure this for themselves and have forgotten these cues that the body gives off, letting the brain know when it needs to be fed and when it's had enough. This is what intuitive eating is going to teach you—how to listen to that inner voice more closely so that you can begin living a life free of food guilt forever (or as close to it as possible)!

Following an intuitive eating plan is literally having to learn how to eat correctly all over again (regardless of your current age).

Intuitive eating is more than just learning when to start and stop eating to stay alive—it's also about accepting your body image and learning to love yourself for who you are. This is probably going to be the most challenging part of this journey, but once you have learned how to accept who you are, you will become happier, feel more fulfilled, and live a life that's more joyous than ever before.

WHAT INTUITIVE EATING ISN'T

It's not another new-age diet or fad to follow. It's a way of life that once adopted will change your outlook on life forever. In fact, intuitive eating has been around since the 1970s and can hardly be called ground-breaking. What is currently trending though is that there is more research and scientific data being gathered and presented in support of intuitive eating.

It's not going to break your bank balance—there are no fancy tablets, meal plans, shakes, smoothies, meetings or other gimmicks that you need to buy to get started (and then be hooked on for an indefinite period).

You get to decide for yourself what foods you'd like to eat, rather than being given a strict dietary routine that can become totally boring after following it religiously for the first week or so.

With intuitive eating, there's no need to count out

calories or measure how many potatoes you're allowed per day. Intuitive eating is completely opposite to a diet. You're actually encouraged to eat the foods that you want, rather than a miserable lettuce leaf and a few carrot sticks as your evening meal!

There is a difference between mindful eating and intuitive eating—although they are similar, they are also different.

THE HISTORY OF INTUITIVE EATING

Evelyn Tribole and Elyse Resch, two well-known and respected dieticians and obesity experts, first wrote *Intuitive Eating: A Revolutionary Program that Works* in 1995 to share their ideas on the philosophy of getting off of diets completely by redefining your relationship with food. They included step-by-step methods that could be used to break habits of emotional eating which we could probably refer to as our comfort food, or binge-eating preferences today. Many saw this book as a revolutionary new way to approach how we eat, although there had already been quite a bit of work on the topic, done by Susie Orbach (1978), who published "Fat is a Feminist Issue," and even Geneen Roth (1982) who wrote about emotional eating habits. All these women were classified as early pioneers in this research and while the term "Intuitive Eating" was only coined in 1995, there were weight management programs founded by Thelma Wayler (1973) known as Green Mountain at Fox Run, which was based in Vermont.

Since then, there have been many more intensive research studies to support intuitive eating, and which we will cover below, but the main emphasis of the entire program was built on the premise that conventional diets don't work and that important changes in personal care are necessary for long-term health.

RESEARCH ON INTUITIVE EATING

In this section we are going to focus on research that has been done since this revolutionary way of eating was discovered—and since the call to "ban the diet completely" was expressed.

The interesting part of this process is that none of these authors or those looking to implement the intuitive eating plan were gym enthusiasts or entrepreneurs, promoting their latest "secret weapon against beating the bulge"; instead, they were all reputable dieticians who had years of experience to back up their theories and methodologies.

We are going to devote the rest of this chapter to discussing some of the studies done since the early days of Evelyn Tribole and Elyse Resch (1995) first putting pen to paper and publishing their book which proved to be the catalyst and game changer on intuitive eating. Up until this point, it hadn't even been given a name. The very first time the words "intuitive eating" were ever recorded and used to name this way of eating was by Tribole and Resch in 1995.

Let's look at a study conducted in a number of universities located in New Zealand, as well as the Ohio State University in the USA. This was conducted by (Barraclough, Hay-Smith, Boucher, Tylka, and Horwath, 2019). For ease of reference, we will refer to this as Study One.

STUDY ONE

The object of this study was to teach more middle-aged women about intuitive eating and taking note of teaching techniques—what worked and what didn't, barriers to success and other obstacles faced in trying to embrace intuitive eating as a new way of life. Findings concluded that women found it extremely difficult to accept that there were no longer any restrictions on the types of foods they were allowed to eat.

This study also discovered the "social and psychological barriers" were the most challenging obstacles to get past.

Part of the educational process was allowing these women to move beyond the standard "good food, bad food" scenario and onto eating whatever they wanted, as and when they wanted, eating when they were hungry and learning to stop when they were satisfied. This proved to be a significant challenge to most within the test group.

The study determined there were definite improvements in feelings of health and wellbeing overall on both a physical and psychological level.

It proved problematic in actually teaching the test subjects what intuitive eating was all about and ensuring they understood it to make full use of it as a new lifestyle. Gaps in training were identified. In a number of studies conducted by nutritional psychologists, it was found that those who had participated in the "Mind, Body, Food" training found transitioning to eating by listening to their bodies far easier than following habitual eating patterns. Those exposed to these interventions (88%), found it to be useful (77%) and easy to use (68%) and said they would recommend it to others (84%)." (David, n.d.)

The test group consisted of only 11 women aged between 41 to 51, of different races, ethnicities, social and economic backgrounds. The results of the above study include the following, which have been revised and condensed for brevity:

INTUITIVE EATING VS DIETING

When dieting (on any form of diet) each of the women described their feelings as being guilt-driven or deprived. They also noted there were consistent feelings of being on a rollercoaster whenever they were dieting conventionally. In contrast, when using the intuitive eating method, they felt as though it was a much healthier approach to food.

"You can have what you want when you want. You just have to pay attention to when it doesn't feel good anymore and stop." (Participant 11).

Additional comments from participants included being able to quieten that voice that screams inside your head, telling you that what you're eating is 'bad for you.'

Others became more accepting of who they were resulting in weight loss almost immediately. Rather than berating themselves, they became more compassionate and self-accepting.

"The most moving part for me was that meditation about accepting your body. I cried. It's a COMPLETELY different way of thinking about your body than the one our culture seeks. Just appreciating the health of your body. I'm a really fit, active

person and I love being active. I really forget to value that." (Participant 5).

Some allowed themselves to now begin eating anything, while others stuck to their rigid 'good food/bad food' mantra.

"If I have a good breakfast and lunch, I could have something naughty for tea and not have to hate myself for it. I've learned not to feel guilty when I do have something that I know is naughty because I've given myself permission to enjoy it." (Participant 4)

Some women embraced this new diet free lifestyle, while others still questioned why they had not lost any weight. They admitted to having more energy and vitality.

HEALTHY FOODS AND INTUITION

This area was not as clean-cut as above as many of the participants battled with where to draw the line on what foods were healthy for them, or simply eating anything until their bodies let them know they were full.

For one of the participants, she discovered that by listening to her body, she was able to feed her body the specific foods it craved at the time—often being the right foods.

DNA OR UPBRINGING?

Many participants felt that they should have been taught the right way to eat by their parents, rather than having to relearn it all over again now. Others felt that we have been conditioned by the world we are currently living in, one that is fast-paced and offers freshly baked, delivered, fast food virtually everywhere you look. While this may be convenient, it does nothing for an intuitive eater.

Because the world has changed so drastically, many of us that fall into this midlife point need to be re-trained to eat correctly, rather than settling for a burger or pizza that can be delivered right to your door. For some this is comfort food when facing an emotional crisis. This is especially when it's necessary to remain strong and focused on getting your mind and your body working together. Taking a stand against the voices in your head and going in search of food that's actually going to make you feel better both inside and out.

Learn how to become more aware of your own feelings towards certain foods. Begin to savor and enjoy them, rather than quickly gulping them down so you can move onto something else you need to tick off your checklist for the day.

CHILDHOOD FOOD PHOBIAS

If you are like me, you grew up in a home where dinner was a family affair at the dining room table. There were no cell phones to interfere with daily conversation and nobody got to leave the table until everyone was finished eating everything! If there was something you didn't like, you had to suck it up and eat it because the alternative was way worse than the taste of spring beans or Brussel sprouts! If you were fortunate enough to have a family dog that you could secretly pass the food onto in a completely innocent way, you may have left the table unscathed. The alternative was spending hours chasing food around your plate with a fork in the hope that someone was going to insist on leaving the table.

The fear of retribution for not eating *everything*, and I mean *EVERYTHING* on your plate at every meal often imprinted on us and has carried itself with us way into adulthood. To this day there may still be certain foods you cannot stomach, and they actually result in a negative emotional connection with that specific food. Being able to detach yourself from this will leave you feeling in control and empowered once more, rather than guilty for feeling the way you do.

REMAINING FOCUSED

Part of the final section of this case study was encouraging and allowing each participant to consistently reassess where they were on their journey and remaining focused on intuitive eating. It was getting them to discover what was deep within them that they could utilize as a means of winning the psychological war against food.

Other members of the control group discovered that it was easier for them to work together with the rest of the members in the group. This was done by being able to connect and network with one another, reaching out when they felt they were about to face a low, or 'fall off the wagon'. They found this camaraderie helpful to provide and receive support from their team—knowing that they weren't the only ones out there who occasionally felt they were losing the war.

Others discovered different techniques to help them overcome their negative body thought patterns and behaviors, also by sharing. This, in turn, helped their mental and psychological well-being and gave many of these women a new lease on life. For many, taking part in this group of test subjects gave them a platform to be of service to one another, discovering that they had a lot to offer others, rather than wanting to be on the receiving end all the time.

FOOD AS A LOVE LANGUAGE

Many of these participants began to realize that there was way more to food than just consuming 3 to 6 meals a day (or whatever your specific needs indicate). They found that approaching the way they viewed food changed their entire outlook towards socializing with others. It increased their willingness to share meals with friends and other family members, without feeling guilty about over-indulging. Better food choices were normally made right at the beginning, preventing unwanted, uncomfortable feelings. By relying on intuitive eating, this experience was once again something to look forward to, rather than dreading holiday get-togethers and the accompanying guilt caused by overeating. Intuitive eating also gave them the power to decide what foods to eat at these festivities—instead of being pressured to dish up something from every plate passed before their eyes. It returned the power of choice as to what to eat and in what quantity.

STUDY TWO

This study consisted of a much larger group of 2,287 younger adults with the average age being approximately 25.3 years old. The main focus of this study was body mass index (BMI) and potential eating disorders that could be associated as a result of intuitive eating (Denny, Loth, Eisenberg, and Neumark-Sztainer, 2013).

Males indicated that they could pick up from their bodies when they needed to eat, as well as how much they needed to eat. The females in this group of studies reported finding it more difficult to know when to eat and when to stop.

In most cases within this study, BMI was not affected at all and those who were able to get their intuitive eating patterns down showed no signs of eating disorders. On the other hand, those who could not tell when to start or stop eating (i.e. they had no idea how to listen to that inner voice within them), were more susceptible to binge eating or chronic dieting.

The same study indicated that long-term dieting is also not a solution. Instead, an alternate healthier way of eating and/or lifestyle is what is needed.

This study also found that being forced to eat everything that's been put on your plate as a child could have much longer-lasting negative effects into adulthood. And so the cycle continues—we demand the same from our children because it's how we have been raised.

Some of the results of this study concluded that we were able to regulate our food intake from a young age (infant), and we continued to do this as a toddler until it was forced out of us. We need to be able to get back to this point again where we can hear that voice that lets us know when we're actually satisfied. We need to listen to it and apply it to our daily lives, not just short term, but as a way of life.

Our bodies know exactly what we need, when we need it, and how to burn what we have stored. Unfortunately, it can't do this if we keep getting in our own way. There has to be a point where we begin to trust our instincts and intuition once more. Allowing that voice to come through and paying attention to what it is saying to us.

WHY ARE WE EATING?

These doctors and professors suggest three reasons why we eat. Think about each of these carefully as you put the next morsel of food into your mouth:

1. Am I eating because I am really hungry?
2. Am I eating because that food smells really good and it's making my mouth water?
3. Am I eating because I'm feeling sad, mad, glad, guilty, or alone?

By being able to identify which of these three categories you fall within, you may begin to decipher what is driving your eating mentally and emotionally right now. You should actually only eat because of the first factor – that of hunger!

HOW DO YOU FEEL?

In his blog (2012), Brian Johnson quotes renowned dietician Marc David as suggesting in his books: "The Slow Down Diet" (2005), and "Nourishing Wisdom" (1994) that we take a closer look at factors influencing us while we eat. Eating out of fear could make us either more fearful or guilty. An example of this would be switching to healthy food to prevent yourself from becoming ill. He also suggests adding another question to the above: how does eating this food make me feel?

Are there psychological factors you may be going through at the moment that may be influencing your current relationship with food? How do you feel about your life in general?

David divides all diets that you could possibly think of into four distinct areas. This could also influence intuitive eating by eating from the place where you're listening to what your inner voice is telling you. These four areas are:

- **Experimental**—don't get stuck on one eating style or set of menus permanently. Every now and again, experiment with exciting new styles of cooking and eating. You may just discover that there are other foods out there that you prefer to eat. These new tastes may excite you and unless you show signs of allergies, you may be able to add entirely new menus to your routines. It can also break down monotonous meals that are actually boring you and potentially robbing you of joy that you should be feeling over mealtimes.

- **Maintenance**—you may be very happy with your current body weight and shape; your BMI may be exactly where you'd like it to be. This is where a maintenance diet is handy. You don't want to do anything extreme by changing too much because this could result in picking up unnecessary weight. At this stage, it's time to batten down the hatches and simply see your diet through. No matter how mundane or boring.
- **Optimizing**—you would be considering an optimizing diet if you were getting ready for a marathon or some other major sporting event where your health and energy levels need to be at their peak. This would result in replacing certain food groups with others. You may need to be loading carbs that you can burn during activity.
- **Therapeutic**—as the name suggests, this style of eating would be especially helpful while recovering from some form of illness or trying to boost your immune system. An example of this would be preparing for a potential flu season by increasing your intake of vitamin C through oranges and guavas. These could be turned into a delicious early morning smoothie to start your day just right.

2

IDENTIFYING THE PROBLEM

"Throw out the diet books and magazine articles that offer you the false hope of losing weight quickly, easily, and permanently. Get angry at the lies that have led you to feel as if you were a failure every time a new diet stopped working and you gained back all of the weight. If you allow even one small hope to linger that a new and better diet might be lurking around the corner, it will prevent you from being free to rediscover Intuitive Eating."

— *EVELYN TRIBOLE*

Just as any good therapist would begin a treatment session, the initial challenge when it comes to intuitive eating is being able to identify food problems you are currently experiencing. It means stepping out of that comfortable space and looking at all the ways you and your body could benefit from learning as much as you can about intuitive eating. What better way to do this than to turn to the experts that got this ball rolling?

KICKING THE DIET MINDSET

Being able to clearly identify where you are with your relationship towards diets and food is the only way to begin to move forward. This is not going to happen overnight—instead, it's a process. It's going to require that you step outside of yourself (or definitely back from your current situation) and analyze the way that you behave and your attitude to food.

This can be much harder than it looks, but there are some ways for you to get started.

DON'T JUDGE YOURSELF

Without being too harsh on yourself or judging yourself in any way, take into consideration your eating habits, behaviors and attitudes. We are normally extremely hard on ourselves when it comes to self-judgment and feeling the need to be perfect in every way. In many instances, this need is what drives our body image.

Ignore the voices of anybody around you with something negative to say concerning your physical appearance. These individuals will always exist. One of the keys to intuitive eating is self-acceptance and learning that you're okay just as you are, rather than having to conform to fit in with what the rest of the world brands as acceptable.

It's what's inside you that counts way more than physical appearance. In intuitive eating, once you've been able to master this challenging phase, your mood, self-image, self-esteem, and self-awareness will each receive the massive boost they need for you to begin to accept yourself as you are. Only then can you begin to become more relaxed and this is when losing weight can begin.

Ask yourself whether you are feeling physically hungry, or whether you need to eat because you are suffering from some form of psychological problem. There are distinct differences between the way these two forms of hunger present themselves.

PHYSICAL HUNGER

Your body is generating signals that it needs food and nutrition at any specific time. Physical hunger is something that occurs biologically within yourself. The symptoms of physical hunger come with physical cues that are given by the body. Some of these cues include your stomach physically growling or rumbling to coincide with feeling empty. You may feel faint and lightheaded or dizzy. For some, headaches accompany this state of hunger. They may even become irritable or show signs of nausea. When physical hunger occurs, the body needs something to ensure it can actually keep going.

If you've been able to confirm that your hunger is physical hunger, then try and rank it on the fullness scale we discussed in Chapter 1. Remember that you're trying to feed your body when it reaches the stage of hunger, rather than starving. Your body will be satisfied with whatever food it's given. This sets it apart from binge eating. When you've eaten something, stop when you are comfortably full, rather than once you've overindulged. Learning to listen to that internal voice can be really difficult at first because you need to drown out everything else you're being bombarded with by the world. Everywhere you look around you, new diets, fads, gimmicks and miracles are being promised as the next best thing to give you the perfect figure, size or weight!

This is the point where you actually need to call "Bullsh*t" on each of these empty promises, because that's exactly what they are. They are there to make money off of you and keep you trapped in a perpetual state of dieting.

KEEP TRACK

It's time to start tracking exactly what you're putting into your body and when. Keep an accurate journal of your eating habits. Begin this food journal without judging yourself. You're aiming to gain a better understanding of the types of foods you're consuming and when. You're also looking for trends in behavior and/or attitude, while not trying to reach any conclusions as to what you're eating or why.

Record as much information in your food journal as possible. This could include things like whether you drank water or a soda; was the soda sugar-free, or an energy drink? Were there specific times of the day where you felt your body hitting a particular "low"?

Working with the sliding scale we've already discussed, record the point that you were at when you started eating, and when you stopped. The ideal is to start when you're feeling hungry and stopping when feeling comfortably full (around 6 or 7), rather than stuffed.

Include how you were feeling on the 1-10 scale. How did you feel afterward?

Being able to review this journal after a few weeks could show patterns or trends beginning to emerge regarding specific foods or food groups that you enjoy eating. You will be able to clearly see whether your liquid intake consisted of fruit juices, smoothies, or energy drinks, rather than choosing water instead (which the body needs daily to be able to function).

IS YOUR HUNGER EMOTIONAL?

Are you eating because you're emotionally drawn to food right now? Do you see food as a means of escaping your current situation? When this hunger appears, what types of foods seem to make you feel better about yourself?

Once you've given into the temptation of "comfort food", how are you feeling about yourself? Do your choices bring on thoughts and feelings of guilt and shame? Additional side effects of emotional eating usually result in low self-esteem because comfort food is seldom healthy food. How many times have you suffered from emotional hunger and thought to yourself, "Ah, I'm off to get myself a healthy salad"? More often than not, it's everything that we should be avoiding, or at least not going all out and overindulging in. Those chocolates aren't really going to make you feel better about yourself. Nor will that tub of ice-cream. Emotional overeating results in you feeling worse about yourself in the long run because you've packed on additional pounds that were unnecessary.

Emotional overeating is a short-term fix to other deep-rooted problems, but the overarching results of unwanted weight gain could leave you feeling even more depressed.

CAUSES OF EMOTIONAL OVEREATING

There are many reasons responsible for emotional overeating. Emotions that could lead to overeating include, but aren't limited to stress, anxiety, depression, losing a loved one, divorce, changing jobs, loneliness, post-traumatic stress syndrome (PTSD), to name just a few. Along with this list, any number of things could trigger a change in the way you feel emotionally. Let's just say that being faced with emotional hunger is like a fuse in a powder keg of dynamite just waiting to be set alight.

Some of them are out of our control, however, our response doesn't need to be to reach for the junk food. Stress is a major cause as indicated, in a letter published by Harvard Health Publishing (2018).

According to research conducted in a survey by the American Psychological Association, approximately 25% of Americans rate their stress levels to be above 8 on a 10-point scale.

The risk factor of the body remaining in a constant state of stress is that the "fight or flight" mode kicks in. Unfortunately, when we're in this emotional state, digestion shuts down, making it more and more difficult for any food consumed to be digested correctly. This "fight or flight" response produces high levels of insulin. This prevents food from being broken down correctly, resulting in weight gain and obesity.

When someone is in a permanent state of stress, additional chemicals are released through the adrenal glands. This is known as cortisol and acts as an appetite stimulant. You can begin to see the problem: you have an increased appetite constantly, but the body's digestive system is in lockdown mode. If you are constantly under extreme stress, all these sugary, sweet "comfort foods" should rather be avoided, or replaced with something that's a healthier option. With all this additional cortisol, feeding the body is necessary, but with the digestive tract affected, processing these foods correctly is a challenge.

COMFORT FOODS

These are all those foods that we reach for or 'crave' when we are having a hard time mentally, physically, or emotionally. It's that packet of chips with the rich dip on the side, it's giving in to the chocolate donuts that call out to you as you do your best to walk past the bakery while en route to another store. It's that tub of chocolate chip ice-cream that has your name on it and calls out to you at the same time late at night. Giving in to any of these foods that have no nutritional value is akin to behaving like a small child with a security blanket. As long as it's there, everything in the world is okay.

Being able to turn to these foods, or anything like them whenever we feel the urge is not healthy for us: this leads directly to binge eating.

BINGE EATING (OVERINDULGENCE)

According to the Oxford Dictionary (n.d.), binge eating is considered to be *"the consumption of large quantities of food in a short period of time, typically as part of an eating disorder."*

It's estimated that this condition affects nearly 2% of the population (Mandl, 2019). Those suffering from binge eating disorder normally present with at least three of these symptoms:

- Eating alone because they feel embarrassed or ashamed
- Eating excessive amounts without feeling hungry
- Eating rapidly
- Eating until uncomfortable
- Suffering from feelings of guilt and/or disgust towards themselves

Because of the above symptoms, people who engage in binge eating find it particularly difficult to come to terms with their body image. This continues to spiral downwards with more guilt and unhappiness every time they go through another binge eating phase. Most find it difficult to break this cycle without some form of therapy or counseling. In many instances, both psychotherapy and counseling are required over an extended period of time before the patient can overcome binge eating.

Research is still thin when it comes to actual causes of binge eating disorders, although much of the research is readily available (PubMed, n.d.). Some causes may relate to both gender and general health. Statistics in the United States indicate at least 3.6% of women will suffer from a binge eating disorder at some stage, while only 2.0% of men will experience the same thing. It's also thought that it could be a characteristic that's passed on genetically.

Other major factors include how we think and feel about our weight and/or body. Whether it's size, shape, or form, if we're not entirely happy with what we look like or feel like, we stand a higher chance of experiencing binge eating at some stage during our lives.

What's interesting about this report is that dieting can be a major trigger for binge eating and if you've suffered from it in the past, there's a strong possibility of relapsing.

RISKS ASSOCIATED WITH BINGE EATING

If all of the information above isn't enough to convince you that binge eating is bad for you, there are a number of potential health problems that could arise from binge eating disorders if left unattended. These include, but aren't limited to:

- Asthma
- Cancer
- Chronic Pain Conditions
- Diabetes
- Fertility Challenges, including polycystic ovary syndrome (PCOS)
- Heart disease
- Insomnia
- Irritable Bowel Syndrome (IBS)
- Obesity
- Stroke
- Type 2 Diabetes

Often those suffering from binge eating disorders aren't even aware that they have this problem. Many of them raid the refrigerator in the middle of the night or make themselves a snack at strange hours when they're supposed to be sleeping. As to whether they are aware of their actions or not, it still constitutes binge eating and is unhealthy for both physical and mental well-being.

EATING BAD FOODS

When it comes to dieting there are always certain foods or food groups that are completely off-limits according to most of the diets out there. Once again, evidence-based findings are identified by what these "bad foods" might include, as well as the reasons why.

While there are many foods that can help you to lose unwanted extra weight, there are others that make losing weight virtually impossible. The eleven foods are identified by Palsodottir as the following:

Beer/other Alcohol—Further studies report that the energy content in 1 gram of alcohol is 29kJ or 7.1 kcal. While in some instances drinking wine in moderation may be healthy for you and assist in losing weight, excessive drinking of other alcoholic beverages could lead to weight gain according to the International Life Sciences Institute, (2013).

There was a direct link to weight gain where heavy consumption of spirits occurred, although this study revealed that further investigation was necessary to identify which specific types of alcohol presented the highest risk. When it came down to it, overindulgence and heavy drinking habits seemed to be the major factor determining potential weight gain and alcohol intake.

Chocolate Bars—one of the biggest contributors to weight gain, with an average-sized bar containing around 200-3oo calories. Most also contain added sugars, oils, and fats. This is usually something that most people add to their shopping carts as they reach the cashier because these are strategically placed there to tempt you to add these items as a last-minute purchase. They are strategically merchandised right where you can be tempted to add them as a final purchase. These chocolate bars are often the number one "go-to" when it comes to comfort food.

If you happen to crave something sweet in the chocolate category, it's best to look for dark chocolate with a high cocoa percentage. As a caveat when it comes to chocolate, always read the labels. You may be shocked by the amount of sugar you're consuming that has no nutritional value whatsoever. All that it's doing is adding to your waistline and leading you straight down the path towards obesity.

Fizzy Drinks—most fizzy drinks and sodas have an extremely high sugar content that isn't processed by the body as food. As a result, no matter how many sugary, fizzy drinks or sodas you consume during the day, your body doesn't feel full at all. Drinking these drinks in large amounts on a daily basis can be hazardous to your health and general well-being. Soft drinks, or any drinks for that matter, are not registered by the brain as food. Although they are loaded with calories, your brain is not processing that you're ingesting any food. It's not registering when you're feeling satisfied, or full. The only way to get around this and being able to win the war against weight is by giving them up completely.

Because your body is made of between 60% and 65% of water, some of which is lost during the day and discarded as waste, perspiration and excreted as urine through the kidneys. Some of it is also lost due to digestion. This water needs to be replaced for the body to remain in optimum condition. Because of this, drinking water is essential for the survival of the body. Water is actually the only liquid that is recognized by the body as a liquid.

Foods with Added Sugar—many products labeled as being "low-fat" are potentially far worse for you because they contain much higher levels of sugar to camouflage the bland taste. Once foods have been processed to be "low-fat" or "fat-free," they lose much of the natural flavor that would be found in fresh produce. When in doubt, it's always a good idea to check out the labels to see actual nutritional values, rather than grabbing products off of the shelves that appear to be "good for you." Examples of these could include many types of breakfast cereal, granola, yogurts, cottage cheese, etc.

Fruit Juices—even the consumption of fruit juices in excess can be a risky habit to get into. While you may believe that those fruit juices that are labeled as 100% pure fruit juice are good for you, realistically, all that they contain is 100% fruit sugar, with none of the pulp (the good part) of the fruit. If none of the pulp is contained in the juice, there's really no point in consuming it.

Some of the best ways to ensure you get the nutrition you need from fruit juices is to go out and buy your fresh fruit from the local store or market and then to process it into a juice yourself. This can be done using a blender which makes certain that all the goodness is left in the juice. It makes for a delicious morning meal replacement, or even a late-night snack, rather than reaching for one of the junk food instead.

High-Calorie Energy Drinks (Caffeine)—hot or cold,

these are a big "no-no." These are readily available in the form of energy drinks and you can virtually find them anywhere. What may seem like a quick "pick me up" when you're needing to concentrate on getting through something or meeting a deadline. These drinks are loaded with caffeine, which is not only addictive but also extremely bad for you. Regarding these energy drinks, it's been reported that "in itself, caffeine is a stimulant, which, if taken on an empty stomach, can make you feel anxious and jittery. Because it's a stimulant it can increase both blood pressure and heart rate, negatively affecting you" (Brown, n.d.).

Energy drinks contain the highest levels of caffeine and are the most dangerous to your health and well-being. If you insist on drinking coffee, try and cut back to one cup a day and drink it black. Signs and symptoms that you may be addicted to your daily fix of caffeine may be suffering from headaches or experiencing irritability when deprived of caffeine. If you get to this point, it may be worth setting an appointment to meet with a health practitioner or dietician for assistance and advice to break your dependency or addiction to caffeine.

Ice Cream—another unhealthy item on the list of foods to avoid. This time because it is high in sugar and calories. The biggest problem with ice cream is that it is comfort food that is easy to consume in vast amounts in one sitting, rather than enjoying in moderation with long intervals in between. Consider limiting the amount of ice cream you dish up for yourself and limit the number of times you can enjoy it during the week or month. As you get into the habit of smaller portions, spread further apart, your body will thank you for it and you won't feel bloated all the time, or consumed by cravings that need to be satisfied.

Pastries, Cookies, and Cakes—because the main ingredients in these are refined flour and sugar, these should be cut back on substantially. It's convenient to stop off for a pie and fries at a local diner at lunchtime, rather than substituting this with a meal that may be healthier for you. Considering all the added sugar that can be found in cakes and cookies, most of the frosting alone is pure sugar, making it difficult for your body to process this amount of sweet food. Once again, a healthier option when craving something sweet is to choose dark chocolate with a high percentage cocoa ratio. This will satisfy your craving and is a much healthier option than conventional chocolate.

Pizza—due to the availability of this as fast food, it's extremely easy to opt for a pizza rather than physically cooking a healthy meal. Pizza is another food that has a base made out of highly refined flour and this combined with all the processed toppings, make it a ticking time bomb! If you really want to treat yourself to pizza, consider making your own at home and choose fresh, healthy toppings – that way you will know what you are eating, rather than accepting what is being handed to you by the pizza joint, where you have no control over where the ingredients have come from, how old they are.

Another problem with pizza is that we overindulge, forcing ourselves to eat the entire pizza in one sitting. If you feel the need to do this, consider scaling back and ordering one size smaller than you normally would. Your body will thank you for making this decision as you won't feel as bloated or disgusted once you've finished the last slice.

Potato Chips and French Fries—the best way to eat potatoes is by boiling them rather than roasting them or deep-frying them. One study on PubMed was conducted between 1986 and 2006 with 120,877 women and men in the USA. Each was assessed over four-year intervals and baselines were adjusted to factor in changes in lifestyle etc.

The results indicated that over each four-year interval an average of 3.35lb was gained mainly as a direct result of eating potato chips. This research concluded its findings to include things like lifestyle changes being linked with the increase in weight gain. This study also showed that most of those with excessive weight gain also consumed alcohol, smoked and did not have a strict exercise regimen.

White Bread—this falls within the scope of refined foods and also contains a lot more sugar than the body needs.

A study conducted in Spain evaluated some 9,267 university graduates for a period of 5-years taking their dietary habits into consideration. After a baseline had been established over 136 different items of food in a questionnaire, changes were monitored and reported annually. Weight changes were recorded specifically surrounding weight changes linked to portions of white bread consumption. By the end of this study, it was found that those who had consumed more than two portions of white bread daily were at direct risk of being either overweight or obese (BMC Public Health, 2014).

TAKING ON NEW DIETS THAT HURT YOU MORE THAN HELP YOU

For anyone who has weight issues or a problem with accepting their body image, dieting is always in the back of your mind and whether you realize it or not, your subconscious is constantly on the hunt for the next magic "fat-melting solution" or "magic pill/potion" that will get rid of the unwanted weight, rolls and flab overnight.

Unfortunately, there are more con-artists out there who are only too happy to oblige and provide you with something that has apparently been tested somewhere in some far off place and promises that it's 100% natural, with no side effects, yet will get rid of all of your unwanted extra pounds overnight. I use the word "unfortunately" at the beginning of this paragraph because thanks to us, these unscrupulous individuals manage to remain in business and even prosper until someone actually does the research into their products and debunks them as another fad or myth!

What you need to understand about diets that are available out there is that there are more than what I could possibly list in the remainder of this book. However, what makes diets and dieting challenging for all of us is that each of us is unique and has unique needs. It's the fact that your DNA is different from my DNA that separates our ability to react the same way to a diet. In addition to this, we may possess other underlying conditions that hamper dieting rather than help it.

Some of these conditions include problems with our thyroid. This could either result in overactivity or underactivity of the thyroid gland. Not only is the thyroid responsible for regulating the metabolism throughout the body but when it's overactive, the following could be experienced:

- Anxiety
- Arthritis
- Diabetes
- Insomnia
- Premature greyness
- Restlessness
- Vitiligo—loss of skin pigmentation

By not understanding everything that is going on in your body, it's simply too risky to get involved with any diet that's not recommended by a medical practitioner. What's even better is to consult with a certified dietician who can assist you with meal planning according to your specific requirements.

WHY WORK WITH A DIETICIAN?

There are a number of reasons to work with a qualified, certified, and registered dietician. The most obvious reason is that they are experienced in this field. Often more so than your normal General Practitioner, or other doctors or therapists. A dietician can work directly with you, refer to your medical history and any recent operations that you may have had. They can take into consideration any chronic medication that you might be on, especially those drugs that have side effects that lead to weight gain. Once you consult with a dietician, you will be surprised by learning how many medicines have weight gain as a possible side effect. If you've been on these treatments for any length of time, it can become more and more difficult to get the body's metabolism back to the point where it's able to lose the weight you have gained.

Just hearing this from a qualified professional can provide us with hope and the knowledge that we can do something about it. A dietician is not going to put you on a "diet" per se: what they normally do is get you eating correctly by focusing on a balanced diet. In many instances, this is exactly what the body needs for its metabolism to begin to function correctly once more.

3

HUNGER IS THE ENEMY

"Instead of indulging in 'comfort food,' indulge in comfort meditation, comfort journaling, comfort walking, comfort talking, comfort manicures, comfort reading, comfort yoga, comfort hugging."

— *KAREN SAMALSOHN*

Probably one of the most challenging aspects to face when on a diet is the hunger pangs that continue to strike. These occur because your body is simply not receiving the right amounts or sources of nutrition necessary for it to function correctly. This is what dieting does. It often starves the body of being able to process the correct nutrients necessary for the body to function properly.

An important factor here is being able to recognize when your body is hungry, feeding it the correct type of foods in the right amounts and regularly enough to sustain and promote good health. Too often when people are on a diet, they allow their bodies to move into a state of starvation before feeding it. This leads to consuming large amounts of food quickly, without actually tasting it and appreciating it for what it is. What this course of action is doing is removing the joy and happiness from the meal and merely replacing this with 'stuffing the food down as quickly as possible.'

HUNGER PANGS AND ROUTINE

The danger of eating in this manner is that hunger is often present at times of the day that fall outside of our 'routine.' This is something that needs to be accepted and honored, rather than ignored because it's the incorrect time to fuel your body.

This is especially true of patients suffering from diabetes—it's better to regulate food intake to 6 smaller meals per day than sticking with 3 meals a day, as this may lead to times where the body is ravenous, to the point that sugar levels drop, and the incorrect foods are consumed in an attempt to give the body what it needs to be able to function correctly.

ARE THERE REALLY CAN'T TOUCH FOODS?

The single most important lesson in this section is that food in itself is not good or bad. You are also not good or bad because of what you do or don't eat. If you are eating intuitively, you could even plan ahead for a treat once or twice a week. This will do a lot to ease feelings of guilt, which then spiral down to feelings of anxiety, depression and stress due to poor food choices.

Eat until you are no longer hungry, and no more.

Listen to the signals of comfortable fullness when you feel you have had enough. As you're eating, check-in with yourself to see how the food tastes and how hungry or full you are feeling. This involves taking your time while you are eating, paying close attention to what the food actually tastes like. To do this we may have to learn to put our knife and fork down during our meal, chew food more thoroughly and drink water as we go.

Most of us focus on getting through a fully loaded plate of food as quickly as possible, without actually spending much time focusing on the texture or taste of the food. We don't spend much time enjoying what we eat or considering what each individual item on our plate tastes like and how it makes us feel! Does it bring us joy? Do we ensure that we remain 'present and in the moment' as we eat? Or are we eating just for the sake of eating? This is where intuitive eating and mindful eating virtually cross paths. It helps us to bring ourselves into the present moment as we enjoy each meal, rather than seeing how quickly we can get through whatever's in front of us so we can move onto the next activity scheduled in our day.

RESPOND TO HUNGER VERSUS ROUTINE

Learn to respond to early signs of hunger that you may be feeling by feeding your body when you are feeling hungry rather than at a specific time. For many individuals, a routine of 3 large meals a day can lead to overeating and gaining weight. If we were raised in a home where you weren't allowed to leave the table unless your plate was completely empty, this could result in weight gain due to overeating.

Learning to feed your hunger as you become aware of it, is much healthier for you to give your body the nutrition that it needs when it needs it. By letting yourself get to the point where you are excessively hungry, you are much more likely to overeat.

DROWN OUT IDEAS OF GOOD AND/OR BAD FOODS

This is another philosophy that's instilled in us from the time that we are adolescents moving into adulthood—the fact that certain foods are good and other foods are bad. In addition to this, you are not defined as either a good or bad person based on the food that you are putting into your body.

Too often young children and teenagers are taught by teachers at schools, magazines and often even parents or peers that 'you are what you eat' and by eating certain foods you are heading down a particular path towards obesity and self-destruction. For really young children, this can cause the early onset of body complexes. Many find it really difficult to get over these beliefs when planted subconsciously from a young age.

While many of these individuals are well-meaning, it's ultimately not their choice to make and they are also not aware of your specific body's needs. When you begin to eat intuitively there's no such thing as one food that's better for you than another. Consider how a diabetic needs to maintain their insulin levels throughout the day in order to function normally. By being forced to stick with a strict diet, this can actually do more harm than good. The foods that have been identified by the diet as being 'healthy' for a normal individual, may prove to be unacceptable for those suffering from underlying conditions. Too many times we deprive ourselves of those things that are exactly what the body needs because we are following a 'diet' to the letter. We don't recognize a craving as something that the body specifically needs. There's a difference between satisfying a craving and overindulgence. One would be wise to be able to identify where the fine line between the two begin and end.

CHALLENGE THOUGHTS THAT TELL YOU OTHERWISE

Whenever you hear a nagging voice in your head that this food should be avoided, or that you need to delay eating at this time because it's not the 'appropriate hour' for you to be eating—challenge these thoughts. Banish them from your mind completely and remind yourself that it's these thoughts that have led you to where you are right now. Unhappy with life and especially unhappy with your body image.

Once you can get these feelings under control and you can allow yourself the freedom of eating when you are hungry, even if the foods are something you would have considered bad before, you will truly be back in control.

While you are challenging your thoughts on whether or not you should eat and when, ask yourself whether your hunger is physically motivated (genuine hunger), or emotionally motivated (there's something deeper going on). If you find that it's emotionally motivated, try and figure out what the emotion is that's behind it and how it's connected to the food(s) you are craving?

Are you eating out of loneliness? Do you feel guilty about something? Are you punishing yourself for something? Observe how you feel about your binge eating session once it's over? Chances are that you are going to be even more unhappy and unforgiving towards your actions and your choices of food!

THE NEGATIVE EFFECT CAUSED BY CULTURAL BIAS

Society has a huge role to play in how we feel about ourselves and the negative body image syndrome that many of us suffer from. As mentioned before, the tabloids and society at large are responsible for the cultural biases that recommend that we should look and behave in a certain way. Unfortunately for society, we are all different and cannot fit into the 'cookie-cutter' mold that they would like us to conform to.

This can be extremely pressurizing for many individuals who feel the need to fall within the parameters of this model. Especially when they are big-boned, heavy-set, have a specific body type and also other pre-existing conditions preventing them from being able to conform to the 'ideal'. It is mainly women who fall into this category, and the failure to be able to conform to the ideal body image as portrayed and/or projected by society, the greater the pressure to do whatever it takes to get there. Namely, diets, pills, fads and exercise programs that don't work for most people.

Many of these diets have not been researched sufficiently, and there is not sufficient medical and/scientific evidence to back up the claims. Far too many individuals spend thousands of dollars annually on trying to achieve the perfect body type or body image they so anxiously desire. When these diets take too long or result in addiction to the "miracle drugs" themselves, the long-term results become even more harmful to those following these diets. Intuitive eating, on the other hand, allows you to decide for yourself what your body wants and what you'd prefer eating, rather than having a diet dictate what you can and can't eat.

SOCIAL MEDIA PRESSURE

Whether we care to admit it or not, we've all got friends on our various social media accounts who seem to have the perfect body and the perfect lifestyle. While they may not intentionally want to rub your nose in it, each time you scroll on your news feed, you can't help feeling totally pressurized by all the ways you don't seem to measure up to them. Each image on their Instagram account makes them look like they've just stepped out of the cover of *Vogue* magazine.

Others are constantly physically active, participating in marathons, cycling events, or other forms of extreme sports. When it comes to comparing ourselves to them, we are maybe not doing ourselves justice. It's easy to see a 'perfect lifestyle' when you're not getting the full picture.

The danger of comparing yourself to others in your social circle is that it could force you further down the guilt and shame spiral. If all that you can focus on is how much you fall short, or fail to live up to the expectations of others, you could easily get stuck in your own head. When you're in this space, you become limited in your ability to recognize those things around you that can bring you joy. Your vision becomes myopic and centered on your short-comings. You become aware of your bulging waistline, the fact that you can no longer fit into your favorite jeans, the fact that you are quickly out of breath simply walking around in a large shopping mall.

This comparison trap is exactly that. It's going to paralyze you where you are and prevent you from physically doing something about it. In truth, we can't all be a size 2. For some of us, there are underlying health issues that limit movement and prevent us from signing up with a gym, getting involved with high impact exercises, participating in marathons, or getting involved in team sports. We need to accept that as much as we are all unique, we also have potential limitations that could be difficult to overcome. As long as you are making an attempt to do something, accept that comparing yourself to others is unrealistic. It can add to feelings of insecurity and poor body image: all those things that you're trying to work through and move past.

As long as you allow your mind to control your body image, especially through comparisons, you will find it more difficult to accept yourself for who you are and make peace with all the positive things your body can do.

4

IT'S ALL IN YOUR HEAD!

"Accept your genetic blueprint. Just as a person with a shoe size of eight would not expect realistically to squeeze into a size six, it is equally futile (and uncomfortable) to have similar expectations about body size. Respect your body, so you can feel better about who you are. It's hard to reject the diet mentality if you are unrealistic and overly critical of your body shape."

— EVELYN TRIBOLE

How you feel about your body image, whether you're pleased with yourself or whether you can't stand looking at your stomach, thighs, or arms—it all starts in your head. Your conditioning is all psychological and once you can identify where and when all of this started, you have a starting point to begin to repair your thoughts and emotions.

MENTAL HEALTH

Mental health is an extremely important factor when it comes to accepting your body image. Without positive mental health surrounding your body, you will be drawn to diets, overindulgence, or even binge eating: it will influence your normal eating habits and possibly even lay the foundations for your children's body image down the line. If you can accept that your body image is all in your own head, you can begin to fix it.

Your negative body image may be as a result of someone teasing you about being a chubby child. While they may have been joking with you at the time, you may have taken their teasing to heart and allowed yourself to be negatively influenced by this name-calling. This may have made you feel negative towards yourself and your body, causing you to begin your dieting crusade in search of the perfect body so that you would never be called a 'chubby kid' ever again.

Learning to accept yourself for who you are is the first step in learning to fix those things about yourself that you don't like very much. Start off by making two lists: a list of those things that you like about yourself, and one of those things that you don't like about yourself. Once you have completed both lists, find someone who you trust, who knows you well, and ask them to be objective while going through each of your lists. You can also get them to add anything else to either list.

They can also cross an item off of your lists and either replace it with something else or give you a reason why they've made the change. You may be pleasantly surprised by how different these lists can actually look. One of the main reasons for this is because we are permanently in our own skin and are too close and judgmental of ourselves. We can't see all the good things about ourselves. Instead, we spend endless amounts of time and energy criticizing ourselves daily for things we either can't change or issues that aren't there to begin with because they're actually all in our heads.

Not accepting ourselves for who we are can leave us filled with low self-esteem which in turn leads to increased levels of stress and anxiety. It's only by accepting who you are, as you are, that you can begin the process of healing and becoming whole again. Once you are able to sort what's real from what's going on in your head, it becomes a little easier to start breaking down some of these mental barriers holding you prisoner in your own mind.

RESPECT YOUR BODY

We are quick to judge and pick up on our shortcomings with our bodies, especially our perceptions when it comes to what we believe is wrong with it—our arms are too short, our toes are ugly, our thighs are covered with cellulite, our butts and stomach are too big and out of proportion. While we are so busy focusing on all of these negative things, we cannot see the wood for the trees, so to speak.

You cannot see your strengths where you perceive weakness(es) to be, or opportunities where before you have only seen failure. Your body is capable of so much more than you are probably giving it credit for. You are probably excellent at so many things, but the harsh judgments you hand down to yourself because of small shortcomings put you at such a disadvantage when it comes to your mental health.

Try and find the beauty in parts of your body. In some instances, you may be so negative about your body image that this is a monumental challenge to overcome.

An example of this is a friend of mine who teaches health, fitness, yoga, spinning, aerobics and aqua-aerobics at a local gym. Since she was a teenager, she has always paid close attention to her health and has been the epitome of fitness. Even now, being super-fit, completing cycle tours and long-distance marathons, she is extremely aware of her own body. Here's someone who has no reason for any negative self-image issues towards her body. She's correctly proportioned, her body mass index (BMI) is ideal, she works out every single day and is toned and tanned in all the right places—yet she hates her body!

She's acutely aware of everything about it, often comments that she wishes she were different and finds faults where there aren't any to be found. I can only begin to imagine how many other individuals are out there who have similar beliefs or feelings towards their perfectly sculpted bodies. This is one of those examples of where a negative body image has been formed and fueled by the mind.

In reality, people would do anything to have her problem of being stuck in a perfect body, yet these individuals see themselves completely differently, maybe as a result of something that happened to them as a child, or an adolescent. Trauma may have occurred that's preventing them from moving forward past this point, and all they can do to control it is to engage in self-loathing and hatred towards their body image and shape.

The right thing to actually be doing if you are in this situation is to start celebrating your body for the many things it is capable of, and recognize just how beautiful parts of your body could be just as they are.

HONOR FEELINGS

Learn to honor your emotions for what they are as and when they arise. Don't give in to using food as a means of coping with any emotions whatsoever. Trust yourself and your body to find other ways of dealing with feelings and emotions—that don't relate to food. There are so many other things that you can be doing rather than binge eating. You need to try and find alternate ways to cope and alternative things to do in the time available that's going to keep you as far away from food as possible. Some ideas are, but not limited to:

- Journaling
- Meeting up with, or calling a friend
- Going for a brisk walk
- Meditating
- Doing crafts
- Trying to learn new skills

The important message to get across when you're feeling this way is to replace the hunger that you're feeling with an activity instead. It's learning to recognize that your hunger is coming from an emotional place. If your hunger is emotion-based, you need to be able to identify the emotion and try and trace it back to where it comes from. Does it have a specific trigger or cycle that it follows? Is it something that occurs daily? Are there specific times of the day when you feel more emotional hunger than others? Is there something else that is causing this emotional hunger to be triggered at this specific time of the day?

TAKE TIME OUT

Something that's important when it comes to switching to intuitive eating is to learn to slow down when eating. This involves not just eating for the sake of eating and getting finished as quickly as possible, but rather learning to savor the food that you have in front of you. It's relearning how to enjoy what you eat, rather than gluttony.

Choose foods that you enjoy and are going to bring you pleasure. Take the time to actually sit down at a dining table to eat your meals, rather than eating your meals on the run. Learn to eat more slowly, savoring the taste and texture of the food on your plate. Take short breaks during your meal, allowing the food to digest properly. This will give your body the time that it needs to let your brain know when you are satisfied. This can't be achieved when you sit with a plate that's piled high and you tackle it like it's the last meal you're ever going to have.

Learning how to eat this way can help your body communicate to your brain once it is satisfied and has had enough. This is the point where you need to physically stop eating. Don't carry on eating because of childhood traditions where you were forced to clean your plate. You will find that eating becomes a genuine pleasure. Discovering foods that you like or don't like will become easier to do because, maybe for the first time since you were a child, you will probably be able to come to terms with each variation of food on your plate.

You will bring the power of eating back into your own hands once more, rather than feeling the need to be force-fed whatever is on your plate. You will rediscover the joy of eating, as well as not having to eat more than your body requires. Your body will also begin to learn that if it should begin to feel hungry, it will be fed with something that it enjoys. This is truly the art of intuitive eating. Less food will be able to satisfy your hunger, and you may find that there are certain new foods that are more appealing to your palate.

5

EXERCISE - THE WAY TO LOOK AND FEEL BETTER

"Even when all is known, the care of a man is not yet complete, because eating alone will not keep a man well; he must also take exercise. For food and exercise, while possessing opposite qualities, yet work together to produce health."

— *HIPPOCRATES*

Instead of embarking on high-intensity body workouts or signing up at the nearest gym to go all out, think about ways to get your body moving initially that will help you feel better about yourself. Contrary to popular beliefs, there's a lot more to exercising than just burning calories that you've consumed.

BENEFITS OF EXERCISE

Finding the right exercise to meet your needs is as important as deciding what foods work for you. The benefits of exercising are as follows, but not limited to:

BALANCING YOUR WEIGHT

Combined with intuitive eating, exercising plays a vital role in helping you control your weight. It also prevents obesity. The best way to maintain your weight is to ensure that the calories you eat and drink equal the energy you expend during the day.

If you are trying to lose weight, the calories consumed as a result of the physical exercise and your daily movement (this includes everything, even cooking and cleaning) need to be higher than the number of calories consumed during the day. Having said this, there's more that needs to be factored in when it comes to wanting to lose weight. Metabolism and any health morbidity should be taken into account. Be kind to yourself when looking to shed some extra pounds. After all, intuitive eating is about loving yourself and accepting your body image for what it is: weight loss is not the goal.

IMPROVING YOUR MENTAL HEALTH

The opposite of exercise is immobility and can normally best be described as lying on a couch or doing nothing particularly productive with your body. This leads to some serious health problems including obesity and heart disease; more importantly it has a negative effect on your mental health as a whole.

Too often, we fail to connect the dots between a lack of physical exercise and a positive mental attitude or our mental health in general. During exercise, the body releases chemicals that improve your mood and make you feel more relaxed. These chemicals are known as endorphins and can help you deal with feelings of stress. They can also reduce the risk of feeling depressed. This is one of the reasons why so many diets insist on a combination of exercise together with the diet.

Exercise also prevents you from focusing on negative things happening around you as you are having to pay attention to physically doing something else instead. According to Gingell (2018):

- Exercise can treat chronic mental health issues.
- Exercise reduces depression.
- Exercise in some cases can be as good as pharmaceutical interventions (this is a huge benefit for those suffering from chronic illness who have been on medication that actually adds to the patient's weight problem, often resulting in drug-induced obesity).
- Exercise can be used to help with anxiety, dementia, depression and even mild cases of schizophrenia.

KEEPING THOUGHTS SHARP

Exercise can also stimulate and release additional chemicals and proteins that improve the functioning of the brain. It can stimulate learning, keep thought processes sharp as well as improve rational decision-making as you get older. Being in better control of your brain and thought processes can help you when it comes to intuitive eating. You will definitely be able to make wiser food choices.

Over 39 different studies concluded that memory

skills and the ability to think clearly were drastically improved for those who exercised regularly (BBC, 2017).

Australian researchers (in the same study) commented that it was worthwhile beginning to exercise at any age: so, if you think that you're too old to begin doing something about your health right now, think again. It was recommended that those who could not take on extremely challenging forms of exercise for whatever reason, try Tai Chi as an alternative.

Findings of this study especially focused on some of the major benefits that could be achieved through regular, consistent exercise, no matter how old the individual or how simple the exercise, the following results were detected:

- Growth hormones, blood supply including oxygen were pumped to the brain.
- Cognitive abilities were improved--some of these included, learning, thinking, reasoning, reading, and reasoning.
- As long as physical exercise was part of the individual's routine, no matter what type of exercise it was, there were signs of improvement.

The ideal recommendation from this study was that regular aerobic exercise was engaged in, to increase the blood flow and oxygen to where it was needed in the body. However, if this wasn't possible, some exercise was better than no exercise whatsoever. Other recommendations included trying to fit at least 150-minutes of aerobic exercise into each week wherever possible.

IMPROVING SLEEP PATTERNS

Regular exercise can help you to fall asleep faster and remain in a relaxed state of sleep for longer. This in turn will help you make better food decisions. Instead of reaching for that caffeine-loaded energy drink or espresso first thing in the morning, you should be waking feeling refreshed and ready to take on a new day without having to rely on anything else to do so.

Dr. Charlene Gamaldo, the medical director of John Hopkins Center for Sleep at Howard County General Hospital, stated following a recent study that "We have solid evidence that exercise does ... help you fall asleep more quickly and improves sleep quality" (John Hopkins Center for Sleep, n.d.).

She further mentions that the time you choose to exercise could impact this ability to sleep properly and that you need to take these into account. For some, exercising too late in the day may leave you too energized, making sleep more difficult.

She recommends (as do the previous studies) that moderate aerobic exercise will likely result in what's termed slow-wave sleep, or deep sleep. This is actually the type of sleep our bodies require to be able to recharge and rejuvenate, getting us ready to face whatever challenges the following day may hold.

She also confirms that exercise can stabilize our moods, allowing the brain to relax to the point where the correct form of sleep is possible.

According to her research, there are two factors which could affect sleep depending on when we exercise during the day:

1. **Aerobic exercises** - endorphins are released which could result in you needing to remain awake. To move past this point, she recommends that you should exercise at least 2 hours before retiring to bed. She clearly states that "the brain needs time to unwind."
2. **Core Temperature** - whenever we exercise, the body's core temperature is raised (similar to when we take a hot shower). The endorphins released send signals to the brain that it's time to wake up. It usually takes anywhere between half an hour to an hour and a half for the body to return to normal temperatures.

Try and figure out what your inner clock tells you regarding exercise, so you are aware of how late you can exercise before trying to get some sleep. This is something that only you will be able to recognize and decide for yourself. Nobody can prescribe exactly what times you should be working out. In the immortal words of Shakespeare's Polonius in Hamlet - "To thine own self be true."

One of the most important things to consider when trying to improve your sleep patterns is that you exercise long enough for your sleep to be positively influenced. Dr. Gamaldo recommends about 30 minutes of aerobic exercise for you to begin to feel the difference in your sleep patterns. She also states that the benefits of exercise will begin to be felt almost immediately.

Find some form of exercise that you enjoy doing; that way you will be motivated to continue with it on a daily basis. Begin slowly at first, especially if you are overweight or obese. You don't want to overdo it on the first day so that you feel as though you never want to exercise again.

When it comes to improved sleep, the returns are almost immediate. You will also begin to feel better about yourself for doing something to make a difference to your own health.

BEGIN WHERE YOU ARE

So, you may be wondering to yourself how you get up off the couch (which is usually your favorite spot to vegetate), and start exercising? The answer is simple—start off slowly. You don't want to go all out immediately because you will burn out quickly or injure yourself, doing your body more harm than good. Remember that you need to be able to respect your body and honor it where it is now.

If you are currently overweight or obese, understand that it took a long time for you to get there, so don't expect a miracle to happen overnight. The excess weight that you're carrying around with you isn't magically going to disappear the moment you begin exercising. Part of being kind to yourself and your body is learning that this is a process and one that's going to take time. Patience is a habit you are going to need to develop and master as part of your 'no-diet' journey into intuitive eating.

Even thinking about where to begin on this road to recovery can be absolutely daunting. These feelings can be fear-based out of self-loathing towards body image. You may not want to appear in public (at a gym) and face up to others whose bodies seem perfectly toned and balanced.

Other reasons for putting off any exercise routine could be out of fear that it's going to be painful to try and push through because you already know that your body is in such bad shape that you don't have the strength to do most of the exercises.

So where do you start if you fall into this category? The American Heart Association (AHA) recommends at least 150-minutes of moderate exercise every week (Timmons, 2016).

This may seem an impossible task, even breaking it down to 30-minutes per day for five days… But, what if this was broken down even further into bite-size chunks that could be managed? Say, 10- or 15-minutes at a time? This is beginning to sound less daunting already. Do what you feel you can manage realistically, without feeling as though you have to climb a mountain. If you manage to get short bursts of exercise in, these all add up in the long run. What's just as important as reaching the 150-minutes per week, is being able to see it through.

Start where you are. Look for ways that you can begin to exercise slowly and build up the strength and stamina necessary to get you going and into a routine. Even if you start and end each day with a brisk walk around your neighborhood. It's definitely a start and before long you will realize that this routine's no longer challenging enough for you. This is when it's time to step it up a notch.

Here are some exercises as recommended by the AHA that you could try and ease into:

1. **Stationary Bike Riding** - These bikes normally have a back-rest, making them ideal for those

who are overweight or obese. Because most overweight individuals battle with their core muscle strength being able to cycle on this type of bike can be the ideal starting point.
2. **Walking** - This is something that's low impact and can be done anywhere. You don't need to pay for it and you don't need any equipment, so even if you're away on business, going for a brisk walk is doable. Begin slowly and as you become fitter, you can increase your pace, distance and duration of your walk.
3. **Water Aerobics** - Very low impact on the body because your body is supported by the water. This has numerous benefits to those who may not be physically able to engage in long walks or cycling. Find a pool that offers water aerobics classes. You may be pleasantly surprised by how refreshing and enjoyable this type of exercise can be.

For someone just starting out, a combination of all three of the above exercises is recommended as they target different muscle groups.

EXERCISE ROUTINELY

As mentioned above, the AHA recommends 150-hours of physical exercise per week in order for you to lose weight or receive physical benefits from an exercise program. Starting is the hardest thing to do. Decide what you most want from your life. Making a decision to begin a simple exercise routine can work wonders for your self-esteem and will yield positive results and long-term improvements to your health and your life.

You are already aware that you're overweight or obese, or you wouldn't suffer from low self-esteem or a poor body image. You're not happy about the way that you look and the only way to make changes is by physically doing something about it. Realizing that taking the first steps towards exercising on a regular basis is one of the few things that are going to help you feel better about yourself is the first step.

You don't need to sign up to that Pilates class or join a gym (unless you want to...). The truth is much simpler: as discussed earlier, the key to being successful is to begin and begin where you are. Do things that are easy to incorporate into your life and your routine. If you have small children, take them for a walk with you in their stroller. You can walk around your neighborhood or walk to a local park. The pace that you begin walking may be slow at first and you may begin to feel your muscles tiring initially. This is exactly when you shouldn't stop because you are beginning to burn those calories.

Some other ways to incorporate physical exercise into your daily routine could be by taking the stairs rather than an elevator whenever the opportunity arises. This doesn't only need to apply to your work environment. Going to a meeting with a client on the 3rd floor? Take the stairs. After a while, you'll begin to feel like you can take on more and more flights at a time without tiring as quickly. Your muscles are starting to be strengthened, so is your stamina and your resolve to keep going.

Some other ways of introducing exercise into your normal, daily routine is by:

- Walk to a co-worker's office rather than sending an email.
- Wash your car on your day off.
- Park your car further away from the shopping mall so you have to walk more.
- Involve your friends and family—explain to them what you're trying to achieve and let them either join you or act as a cheerleader to your exercising cause.
- Get involved in classes that require exercise: try YouTube videos for Zumba or other classes, and follow these routines in the comfort of your own home.
- Take your dogs for a walk/run every day.
- Sign up for physical activity groups—volleyball, water polo, dance, hiking, kickboxing, figure 8 dance classes.

If you're just starting out in your quest to become physically fit, it may be worthwhile to try out a couple of different classes to see which resonates with you, before signing up and committing time and money.

Groups are a great way to go because the participants often act as cheerleaders to keep each other motivated.

TRACK YOUR PROGRESS

Keep a journal that can track your progress. This could include the physical activity you were engaged in, the amount of time you spent doing it, and possibly the way that it made you feel at the end. An example of this would be:

[Date][Physical activity engaged in][How long or how far][I feel...]

Nobody is suggesting that you make a novel out of this, rather keep a simple diary to monitor what you are doing. After a short while you should begin to notice that during the same period of time, you are able to achieve more. This is an indication that your body is beginning to get stronger and your stamina is improving at the same time.

An example of this would be if you were to begin walking. Initially you may only be able to walk for 10 minutes in a day without feeling uncomfortable or tired. After a month of regular walking, you may notice that you've been able to increase the amount of time that you're walking to 20 minutes and you've more than doubled the pace and distance.

You could use apps that you could download onto your phone that can help you calculate how many steps you walked for the day. Begin by setting smaller goals for yourself and increase these incrementally over time. As you reach each of your goals, celebrate each achievement. Once you've done so, set a new target so that you keep yourself motivated towards pushing yourself further constantly. Goals achieved need to be rewarded - try not to attach this reward to food though! Find some treat that you really want and reward yourself as you reach each of your fitness/weight goals. Replace what used to be a food-based reward with something else. An example of this could be booking a massage, buying a new item of clothing, treating yourself to a movie at the cinema.

These are the small victories that you should be aiming for. Some other tools that you could add to your arsenal against your negative body image are things like a tape measure, a scale, and even a mirror. Your clothes may give you another indication that you're beginning to shed some weight.

In your fitness journal, record how you are beginning to feel about changes you're experiencing, especially towards your body image.

PUT THE FUN BACK INTO EXERCISE

You are likely to get bored easily by repetitive exercises over a long period of time. You can overcome this by trying to bring the fun factor back into exercising. Apart from listening to music or watching TV while you work out, mix up your activities. Set up an exercise schedule that has some variety and try making changes to the schedule so that you aren't doing the same exercises each day.

Consider exercises that can be done year-round, taking the weather into consideration. If it's raining, find exercises that can be done indoors. The main point of getting into an exercise routine is being able to stick with it so it has a positive impact on your health and your weight. This is vital for a positive body image.

The main aim of exercising is to get the body moving, the blood flowing and to help you feel better about yourself. If the added benefit to this is weight loss, then this is a bonus. You are trying to ensure that your physical and mental health needs are taken into consideration.

Here are a number of other ideas that can easily be incorporated into your routine to spice things up a bit:

- **Dance like no-one is watching**. Being self-aware, especially when it comes to having a negative body image can be one of the toughest battles you will ever have to face when exercising. At some point, you need to just stop caring about whatever the rest of the world thinks and realize that you are doing this for you. Show up for yourself and work through the gamut of emotions that will come as you begin to become more physically fit. Don't listen to what anybody else has to say. Their opinions are not important: your health is!
- **Don't procrastinate.** It's easy to hit the snooze button in the morning and roll over going back to sleep rather than going for a walk, run, or engaging in your chosen exercise routine. This is where you need to be strong mentally and make a decision that no matter what happens you will stick with it. Decide that you aren't going to place your health on the back-burner any longer - instead, you are going to regain control over your life.
- **Find your reason.** Rather than exercising because you hate the way you look, use self-esteem, self-awareness and self-care as reasons to motivate you onwards and upwards. If you are battling with low self-esteem, do it for a loved one. This could potentially be for your spouse or your children. Set a goal that includes them as part of your reason for wanting to be more physically fit and healthy.
- **Try weights on for size**. A popular myth in

health and exercise circles is that if you are overweight you need to get cardio going first, before moving onto weight training. This is not true. You can begin with weights in the comfort of your own home. Another benefit of choosing to add weight training to your routine is that it works much quicker than cardio on its own. Training with weights will allow you to quickly notice that you are becoming physically stronger. As this happens, you will become more motivated to continue working with weights. Weights can also be adjusted according to how far you're ready to push yourself. You can add or subtract weights until you feel comfortable.

- **Sign up for a walk-a-thon or a race.** Look for those that have short distances that you know you'd be able to handle. Ask a friend to join you or involve your partner and your family. They are ideal motivators. Mark the date down on the calendar and place this somewhere prominent where you'll see it every day (like the fridge). You can often find charity events of this kind. Most of these are advertised on social media such as Facebook. All you need to do is commit to attend and put the work in to prepare to participate.

6

HOW DO I ACTUALLY EAT INTUITIVELY?

"Having a healthy relationship with food means you are not morally superior or inferior based on your eating choices."

— *EVELYN TRIBOLE*

HOW TO EAT INTUITIVELY

According to Rumsey (2017), there are five specific tips that she shares to improve the relationship we have with food. It all begins with getting rid of the misconception that certain foods are better than others, and that depending on what you eat you should feel guilty about it. Her five tips are to:

- **Forget about diets (all of them)** – all diets do is make you feel guilty about yourself and even worse about your body image. This is the antithesis of what you're trying to achieve. You want to begin to feel better about yourself. If you wanted to feel bad, you could go back and join all of these diet groups where you need to weigh yourself every couple of days, count how many calories you're eating within a day, etc. If you've made friends with these people via Facebook or LinkedIn and are watching videos on YouTube or listening to podcasts as to what you should be doing and how you should be doing it, I have two simple words for you —STOP IT!

You can replace these with those that promote anti-diet living instead. Some of these are listed below with the links in the reference section:

- Immaeatthat blog
- Rachael Hartley Nutrition blog
- The Foodie Dietitian blog
- The Real Life RD blog
- Food Psych Podcast
- Love Food Podcast
- Nutrition Matters Podcast
- The Nurtured Mama Podcast

- **Understand and use the Hunger/Fullness scale** – we've covered this in previous chapters, but this scale can be quite challenging to come to terms with initially. The biggest challenges occur in being able to tell when you are actually feeling hungry (when the correct time it is to eat), and when you've had enough to eat (when you are satisfied but not overstuffed).

Getting this balance right takes time to master. It's about learning to eat slower, to actually enjoy the food(s) that you are eating when you are eating them. It's also about taking regular breaks during your meal to analyze how 'full' you are feeling at the time. This is so that you get to recognize when you are feeling comfortable and satisfied, rather than uncomfortable because you've overeaten. This is the most challenging part of intuitive eating.

Discovering exactly how you feel in terms of fullness or satisfaction and then honoring these feelings by putting your knife and fork (or spoon) down. It's moving past that old mentality of having to eat everything on your plate simply because it was placed there.

- **Eat exactly what you want to eat** – the reason why this pointer is so powerful is that it breaks the 'diet' mentality completely. It no longer restricts you with those foods that you can or can't eat. You can throw out the list of all the things that you have up to this point considered to be 'bad' for you. Suddenly the physical 'craving' of certain foods is removed because the barrier or ban on eating them has been lifted. Have you ever been on a diet where you weren't allowed 'ice-cream' and found yourself craving it multiple times a day? Eventually, at some stage you would cave and go on an all-out ice-cream eating binge, only to hate yourself for doing so the next day!

If you think about this psychologically—when there are no barriers to hold you back regarding those foods that you can or cannot eat, the pressure of having to fill the empty void of craving is gone. That ice-cream may be a small treat for one day of the week or once every two weeks. You aren't physically removing it from the equation and placing labels on foods—making some good and some bad!

PRACTICE MINDFUL EATING

Rumsey (2017) continues by suggesting that you practice 'mindful eating' – this is where you pay close attention to what you are eating, where you are eating (your surroundings), and what each mouthful of food physically tastes like. It's like starting a taste bud revolution and discovering the taste of foods as if you were eating them for the very first time.

To eat mindfully you need to be able to slow your eating patterns down considerably. Physically taking the time to chew each mouthful of food properly. Allowing your taste buds to work their magic. What does the texture of the food do to your mouth? How does the food make you feel?

Mindful eating involves physically sitting down at a table and ONLY eating. It's not multitasking by eating in front of the TV, or computer. It's also not grabbing your meals on the run while you rush out of the door, late for that business meeting or appointment and you have your briefcase in one hand together with the car keys and a croissant in the other that you can gulp down in the car on the way. It's also definitely not stopping through a fast-food drive-through on the way home because you're exhausted from your day and you just know that cooking is the last thing you want to do once you get home.

When you master mindful eating, you'll begin to notice when you're hungry, and also when your body is satisfied. You'll treat your body with more respect as you take your time with each meal, focusing on the food itself and the way that it's making you feel. This will replace current unhealthy habits that you have with food at the moment, with ones that are going to be more beneficial to you in the long run.

CHALLENGE THE FOOD POLICE

Her final tip is to challenge the 'food police' running around in your head! This is those voices that keep challenging you with what you can and can't eat. These voices have been around for a long time. For many of us, most of our lives (or at least since we were teenagers and began all these see-saw diets).

How can you recognize the food police? Easy—whenever you hear a nagging voice in your head telling you that you shouldn't have eaten this or done that! These are the voices that make you feel guilty and inferior. Sometimes they can bring self-loathing and guilt with them – telling you that you are fat and/or ugly and nobody will ever be able to love you!

We mentioned keeping a journal and a logbook for your exercise. Another journal may be a good idea to begin tracking these negative internal thoughts that you have about yourself. Whenever you recognize any of these thoughts entering your mind, write them down. You can then begin to pull them apart and physically analyze them. Where do they really come from? Are they real? What is the pay-off for this kind of thinking? Make this journal an active part of your day and go through it often. You may discover that certain patterns begin to emerge that are linked specifically to either a specific time of day or a particular food. Once you discover this, they become easier to face head-on and deal with one at a time.

ONLY YOU CAN DECIDE

Up to this point, you may have thought that you have no control over what you eat, how much you weigh and your self-image. This is simply NOT true! If anyone has the power to change anything about yourself, it's you and only you. You are the one who needs to decide and make the necessary adjustments to meet your own specific needs.

In intuitive eating, the main rules are to eat only when you're hungry and to stop when you're feeling satisfied (rather than stuffed). It's using your 'intuition' or 'common sense' to do so. While this sounds fairly easy to do on paper, in reality it's way more difficult because finding and listening to what your intuition is telling you to do is often drowned out by the voices of the world.

The glossy magazines, billboards, social media advertisements, television, movies and everything else out there want you to feel bad about not having the 'perfect look.' What is the 'perfect look' for you anyway? You know your body, you know your bone structure better than anyone, therefore it makes perfect sense that this whole 'perfect look' thing should be left in your own hands.

It's time to stop listening to what everyone else around you are saying and doing. It's time to begin ignoring what the world wants and figure out what's going to make you happy. Once you've managed to do this for yourself, you will begin to feel more in control of where your life is headed.

RECOGNIZE AND FEED YOUR HUNGER

Hunger plays a key role in intuitive eating. It's the time that you should be giving your body enough nutrients, energy, and food that it needs in order to survive and thrive. There are two different types of hunger though and you need to be able to tell them apart.

Physical hunger happens naturally throughout the day at regular intervals. Depending on your body type, your physical health and any other underlying conditions which you may be suffering from, this hunger may need to be fed anywhere between 3 to 6 times daily.

If your hunger is connected to your emotions, try and find another outlet or way of dealing with whatever's going on with you. Identify the emotional trigger and attempt to work through it. This type of hunger is easy to fuel with comfort food (which is almost always exactly what you should avoid). Emotional hunger is what leads to binge eating and it's this that packs on the pounds because emotionally you're more inclined to retreat, rather than taking any form of action. It's this hunger that causes you to retreat to your bedroom with that tub of pistachio ice-cream and a spoon—leaving you feeling totally guilty in the morning!

Find ways to overcome emotional issues by choosing to be physically active instead. Get out, breathe in some fresh air and go for a brisk walk: it's better than sitting around feeling sorry for yourself. Most of all, be kind to yourself. Accept that you are feeling something that needs to be worked through. Journaling can often help to work through these issues as well.

CHOOSE FOODS WISELY

With all of your food choices, try and include as many fresh fruits, vegetables, and other staple foods as possible into your diet. This is normally where we fall short. We fill ourselves with too many processed foods that have no real nutritional value and can't satisfy physical hunger. Aim to include as many fresh foods as possible in your daily menu. Consider foods that are seasonal, as nature has a way of providing us with all the nutrients we need when we need them. There's a reason why certain foods are seasonal. Citrus grows mainly in the cooler months. Being rich in vitamin C, these fruits can help strengthen immune systems and help prevent colds and flu.

This may require doing some research but try and find those fruits and vegetables that are seasonal. Nuts, legumes, tubers and even meats are required to be balanced in our diets. Find what works for you. As long as the body is receiving all the nutrients it needs to survive and thrive. Fresh is always better than processed or frozen wherever possible.

BENEFITS OF INTUITIVE EATING

According to Jennings (2019), some of the major research-based benefits of intuitive eating are:

Those following intuitive eating plans have more positive attitudes towards lower body mass index (BMI) and weight management versus weight loss. This was according to studies published in PubMed (n.d.)

Improved psychological health, self-esteem and quality of life. This occurred because they had a better self-image making them less susceptible to anxiety and depression. In addition to this, these women were inclined to maintain the distance once following an intuitive eating plan. This was completely opposite of a regular diet mentality according to a study conducted by Schaefer and Magnuson (2014).

This same study also showed that following this kind of program led to long-term behavioural changes when it came to eating.

A third study completed by Ricciadelli (2016) indicated that those women who managed to master the art of intuitive eating were far less likely to display other eating disorders.

While much research has already been done on intuitive eating to date, there is still much that needs to be done to support these findings and more.

7

MY 5 STEP PROCESS TO SUCCESS

"Your body needs to know consistently that it will have access to food—that dieting and deprivation have halted, once and for all. Otherwise, your biology will always be on call, ready to avert a self-imposed food deprivation."

— *EVELYN TRIBOLE AND ELYSE RESCH*

In their bestselling book, Tribole and Resch challenged every major belief that dieting up to this point in history had claimed to be. In this book, they focused instead on providing a solution for those individuals who had tried diets and failed hopelessly. They provided a 10-step plan to challenge old belief systems and introduce new methods of thinking.

In an attempt to simplify their process even further, I'd like to provide you with the following five steps to get you motivated towards making healthy changes in your life that can have a lasting impact. These steps are not merely a fad or a phase to be adopted for a few weeks, only to be abandoned at the first sign of failure. Instead, they are meant to keep you motivated in building genuine life-altering habits that will become a lifelong commitment towards permanent change.

STEP 1: HOUSTON, WE HAVE A PROBLEM

Identify that you have a problem with consistent dieting, a poor body image, low self-esteem, or addiction towards trying on every single new diet or fad that comes onto the market. As with anyone suffering from any form of addiction, the first step in the recovery process is admitting to the fact that you have a problem in the first place. Own it and accept it.

- Recognize what this addiction is doing to you.
- How is it affecting you, mentally, physically and emotionally?
- How is it affecting your relationships with others?
- How long have you been unhappy with your body image?
- Is this preventing you from living your best life?
- Identify every negative sub-problem that's accompanied the diets.
- How much money have you spent over the years? (This could be on anything from gym memberships to lotions, potions, diet pills, and equipment including trainers, sweats, etc.) This financial figure should be enough to send you reeling!

- How much time have you wasted preparing all these diet meals and concoctions?
- How much time have you wasted reading labels while shopping and then paid twice as much on items because they say 'low-fat' or 'sugar-free,' only to discover that they're actually loaded with more sugar than the normal product (artificial sweeteners)?

STEP 2: ACCOUNTABILITY

Accept accountability for your own life. For your thoughts, feelings, and emotions. Analyze and recognize where your thoughts, feelings, and emotions are coming from when referring to your body image. Where did it start? Is it real? How has it affected you over the years? The key to this step is doing a deep dive into your own head. You'll be surprised by just how much of your low self-esteem, poor body image, frustrations, and emotions have built up over many years. You can probably trace the roots back to that one instance where that person happened to pass the comment about you being a "chubby kid."

Finding the origin of your belief system can help you to figure out what you need to be doing to heal yourself. Or at least where you can begin to challenge these beliefs. When we are young, it is easy to accept whatever we are told, especially if we were raised in an environment where you were forced to eat a specific way. These formative years can potentially shape us into dysfunctional adults.

You may have become addicted to dieting during your

younger adolescent years—not quite sure how to deal with body changes during puberty. Step 2 is all about getting to the root of your dieting dilemma. Discovering where it started. Only once you can recognize the beginning, can you begin to unravel the chords that are keeping you so tightly bound to constantly being at war with your body image.

STEP 3: DITCH DIETS FOR GOOD

We've learned from Evelyn Tribole and Elyse Resch (1995) that diets don't work and that it's way more important to listen to what your body is telling you. The people who managed to get off of the dieting merry-go-round are much happier, healthier individuals. They no longer count calories or try to figure out how much extra time they need to spend working out at the gym because they enjoyed a small slice of cake at the office celebrating a colleague's birthday!

Intuitive eating is all about recovering from yo-yo dieting and learning to become more intuitive by listening to what our bodies tell us about ourselves. It's figuring out what foods we prefer. It's about learning to slow down and appreciate our food for what it is, nutrition and fuel that the body needs to survive and thrive.

STEP 4: EMBRACE INTUITIVE EATING

Intuitive eating is not intended for the body to specifically lose weight, although weight loss may come as a natural by-product of eating correctly. Instead, it's about creating a positive body image for yourself so that your self-esteem is enhanced, and you are treating your body on a holistic level.

Getting into the habit of intuitive eating could assist you to shed pounds because the body is no longer in 'starvation' or 'stuffed' modes, which is exactly what many of these diets do. They create environments of either 'feast or famine' and the body is never certain where it stands. This is what leads to fatty deposits building up in the body as it stores food as a spare supply because it's not sure when it will be fed again! This is one of the biggest challenges and experiences that the body physically undergoes during a diet.

In intuitive eating, there will always be food there when the body feels hungry, and it will be able to have enough food until it's satisfied. It no longer needs to store extra fatty deposits—this is what could potentially lead to natural weight loss with intuitive eating. Accept and understand that intuitive eating is NOT A DIET!

STEP 5: IN IT FOR THE LONG HAUL

Accept that you need to give intuitive eating a chance to work and that it's not going to make major changes to your body overnight. Yes, you will certainly feel the benefits of being able to eat when you are hungry. The challenge is learning to read the cues that are going to tell you when to stop eating. This is where you need to become patient and eat slower, savor each mouthful—chew your food slowly. Enjoy each mouthful as if it were the last.

Commit to seeing intuitive eating through for at least 90 days. Avoid being tempted to hop back onto the next new dieting craze, just because it's there. Practice the techniques that have been included in the previous chapters, as well as those that follow. Your goal is to learn to love yourself and make peace with the relationship that you have with food. Remember to stick with your notes and keep on journaling on how eating intuitively is making you feel about yourself. For example, you can use these questions as prompts for daily journaling.

- How are you feeling about your relationships with others as a result of intuitive eating?
- Are you feeling more comfortable in your own skin?
- Is it easier for you to accept your current body image?
- What else has this journey taught you?
- How can you ensure that this becomes part of your life moving forward?

8

STOP BLAMING YOURSELF

"The Dieter's Dilemma is triggered by the desire to be thin, which leads to dieting. That's when the dilemma unfolds. Dieting increases cravings and urges for food. The dieter gives in to the cravings, overeats, and eventually regains any lost weight. He is back to where he started, with the original weight —or higher. And once again the dieter has the desire to be thin ... and so another diet begins. The Dieter's Dilemma is perpetuated and gets worse with each turn of the cycle. The dieter is heavier and feels more out of control with eating."

— *EVELYN TRIBOLE*

WHY BODY IMAGE?

Up to this point, we have been focusing on many of the reasons why individuals find the need to follow the latest diet trend. It may surprise you to hear that the number one factor that leads to any form of dieting is how we perceive ourselves and our body image. This is what we see when we look in the mirror. Our reaction to this image may be realistic, or it can be flawed. It's this flawed image that leads us to dieting, even from a young age.

We have an image of what we 'should' or 'shouldn't' look like on the basis of what society is telling us, what our parents are telling us, what our peers are telling us or a variety of other reasons. This is not to say that any of these reasons are true and correct. Breaking free from the bonds of body imaging is the aim of this chapter. I hope that you will gain greater understanding and appreciation for your body as it is now and learn why dieting is not the answer to changing the way that we feel about our bodies.

THE BODY IMAGE CONCEPT IS FLAWED

Statistics reported by The National Eating Disorder Organization (n.d.) indicate that awareness and concern for body image can begin in girls often as young as 6-years old! Girls between six and 12 are already worried that they're too fat. This is according to the publication by Thomas F. Cash and Linda Smolak entitled "Body Image, Second Edition: A Handbook of Science, Practice, and Prevention." (2011). This leads to looking for solutions by beginning to diet from such a young age. Some children turn to extreme diets and destructive behaviors that can range from smoking to taking laxatives, eventually developing eating disorders. Some unfortunately even go as far as developing anorexia nervosa or bulimia as they search for acceptance from their peers. Even the children who don't go on to develop serious issues become addicted to the diet mentality from an early age and unless the cycle is broken, this will follow them throughout their entire lives.

The only way to break this cycle is by learning to accept and love your body exactly as it is. It's learning to be grateful for the things that your body is able to do. How it supports you and carries you throughout the day. How you are able to move in a certain way, unrestricted and unhampered. It's being able to express gratitude and celebrate what you have, that many other individuals possibly don't have.

THE PERFECT BODY IS A FANTASY

Who or what determines what the 'perfect body' looks like? Is it a particular proportion? Facial features? Body shape? BMI? Is this decided by society? Peers? Parents? Or is it all in the mind? Should this decision actually be left to anyone other than yourself? Surely the perfect body or ideal body image is when we can get to the point of being comfortable in our own skin. Rather than benchmarking ourselves against celebrities, online influencers, or those lean, mean, toned 'models' promising you instant results if you just buy that shake or follow that diet. This is why buying into the whole dieting mentality doesn't work.

There are only so many people who are born with the perfect genetic makeup and body metabolisms that can process the food that they eat at a rapid rate, ensuring that they always look slim or lean. For others, they really work hard to get there and maintain a strict lifestyle of exercise and balanced food intake. This is completely different from following a strict 'diet' regimen to get to where they want to be.

They aren't sacrificing foods to stay fit—they've balanced their food intake according to what they are burning off during any given day's exercise, whether this is at the gym, running, swimming, playing golf—you get the idea!

They are not restricting their meals in any way: they have just learned what works for them and so can you. They are not fanatical about how they look, they are more interested in how their bodies can function.

WHEN DOES IT BECOME A DIET?

Any style of eating that restricts you from certain food groups or limits your intake of calories, carbohydrates or requires that you cut out other foods such as proteins, fats, carbohydrates or even wheat, should be classified as a diet and must be avoided at all costs. The body needs everything to function at an optimal level and the natural reaction to being told that it cannot have a certain type of food is that the body will 'crave' that specific food even more.

Rather than following all of these diets, from Paleo to Weight Watches, all the way to Intermittent Fasting, it's better for your body image and yourself to get rid of any and all siren calls that promise miraculous results within a matter of days.

ACCEPT YOUR BODY AS IT IS NOW— CELEBRATE IT

Accept your body for what it is now and learn to practice self-love instead. This should replace self-loathing because this is what is leading you to your poor body image in the first place.

If you're a mother who's now carrying around some extra weight that you haven't quite lost since you've had your children—celebrate this! You've had the opportunity to bring new life into this world. Celebrate each milestone that your children reach and think of the joy that they bring into your life daily.

If you have the use of your arms and legs, celebrate this and be grateful for everything that you can do with your limbs. Be grateful that you're able to walk daily and keep your body moving. If you can still bend and stretch and are supported by your spine—be grateful and celebrate all the things you can do. If your spine allows you the simple pleasures of picking up your children, or doing daily chores, being able to reach for things in supermarkets or stores while shopping—consider those suffering from bone deterioration that are unable to do these things anymore. Think of those now limited as to how far they can walk each day, or possibly even being confined to a wheelchair.

If you can see and hear and smell—be grateful for these abilities to be able to appreciate the beauty of the world around you.

While each of the above may seem to be obvious things our bodies can do for us each day, how often do we actually take notice of them? Do we accept and appreciate what we are able to do, or are we so focused on our perceived faults and flaws that we can't see what we already have?

Take out your journal and begin to write down all the things that your body can do for you right now—you'll be surprised at how long the list is, and how liberated you will begin to feel afterward.

FORGET THE FANTASY

Fantasy, perfectly shaped and proportioned bodies that look like they have been sculpted by an artist are far and few between. Those that are have possibly taken years of professional coaching and training to get there. Believe me, no matter what anyone says in any diet book, article, feature, advertisement, or blog—there's no new fad or gimmick that hasn't been kicked around the block a few times for decades before (in some instances even for centuries).

Anyone promising you instant results is a fraud. There's no such thing. Learning to eat correctly and getting your body moving is the only way to go, and you are the only one who can get intuitive eating mastered effectively.

You know what your body is saying to you and you need to follow the signs and cues that it provides you with. Be prepared to move more than you've done in the past, if you want to begin to see results, but remember that intuitive eating is not a diet! The promise of weight loss isn't attached to this plan. It could potentially be a by-product of learning to listen to what your body is telling you.

Remember that people come in all shapes and sizes, life has always been that way. We cannot all resemble models on the cover of glossy magazines (nor should we want to). You need to recognize sales and marketing ploys, especially around the dieting industry to be exactly what they are - lies that we've been fed to believe we need their products to become acceptable.

LET GO OF THE NEGATIVES

Whatever negative body image thoughts you've been holding onto—it's time to let these go and let them go for good. This is actually way more difficult than it sounds, purely because most of us have been raised with a negative mentality towards our bodies from a young age.

Your current negative thoughts surrounding your body image need to be banished.

But how do you achieve this when your negative thoughts can become totally overpowering at times? Get that journal out once again and write down at least ten things you like about yourself. Whenever you find your mind wandering off to the 'dark side' of negative body image, go back over this list again. You may even want to print this list out and place it somewhere prominent where you can read it daily. This will help it become a mantra to your daily living.

Just as we've dealt with the 'food police' in a previous chapter, where you're able to ward them off rather than paying them any attention, you can follow the same trend whenever you are faced with negative voices that tell you that you have imperfections with your body. (As a sidebar

—even those who have the so-called 'perfect bodies' aren't 100% happy with how they look).

Another valuable tip is to see yourself as a full individual—that is, more than just what your body looks like from the outside! There are a lot of people out there who have bodies that look perfect, yet inside they are horrible people! Beauty is more than skin deep; it takes your character and personality into consideration as well. Never forget that!

Monitor social media messages—what are they really saying? And, more importantly, are they real? Call them out whenever they're fake. Remember that you determine what you choose to believe and listen to—not social media or any media for that matter.

Be kind to yourself. We live in a world that can be harsh, judgmental, and dominated by plastic people. Take the edge off of some of this hurtful mentality by being kind to yourself. So you've had a rough day at the office, instead of aiming directly for that tub of ice-cream and a spoon to comfort you—stop and buy yourself some flowers instead. They will last longer than the ice-cream and beautify your surroundings, making you feel better about yourself.

Be of service to others—it's true that when you are serving others you can often lose yourself. Your own imperfections and shortcomings can easily become swallowed up while doing something kind for someone out there who is in greater need than yourself. If you're not sure where to begin with this, look at contacting animal shelters, homes for abused women or children, or consider visiting the elderly in local hospitals or assisting community projects to clean your parks, schools, or beaches, all are worthwhile pursuits.

BANISH THE BLAME GAME

Whenever we begin to gravitate back to negative body image, we begin blaming ourselves, our parents, our loved ones, or anyone else who happens to be in the way for allowing ourselves to get like this—even that chocolate cake! Whether it's genetics or choices we choose to use as a hook, we have an innate desire to lay the blame somewhere, and most of the time it falls directly back on our own shoulders.

The moment this happens, a negative spiral begins moving us downwards and closer towards a host of eating disorders. This happens because someone needs to be held responsible for allowing us to become this way. We see our bodies differently. This image is often distorted and removed from reality and this distortion is often the cause of eating disorders.

EATING DISORDERS

Eating disorders can range from physically abstaining from food—starvation, to binge eating disorders and a whole host of others in between.

Anorexia Nervosa

One of the most dangerous of all eating disorders. It starts out with some type of 'harmless' diet and ends up with total starvation. Those with anorexia cannot see themselves as skin and bones. Instead, whenever they look in a mirror, the image that's projected back at them is someone who's morbidly obese! The sad truth about anorexia is that most cases take years to recover with extensive therapy and counseling, or they could result in life-long serious medical issues or even death.

Bulimia nervosa

Bulimia nervosa is another serious eating disorder that claims many lives each year. Although it is similar to Anorexia nervosa, the main difference is that those with bulimia actually eat and then physically make themselves ill by sticking their fingers down their throat. The danger with bulimia is that gastric juices pass back through the esophagus often causing permanent damage. These are serious eating disorders and if you have the tendency to engage in this self-destructive behavior to try and lose weight, please seek help in the form of professional counseling.

Bulimia can also cause death in extreme cases, due to cardiac arrest caused by the stress that the body is placed under while it lacks the necessary nutrients to function correctly.

Neither anorexia nor bulimia should be taken lightly. For many suffering from bulimia, laxatives can be used as a form of getting the body to physically purge whatever food has been consumed.

Opting for a self-administered colon cleanse in the hopes of losing weight can rob the body of the very nutrients, fats, carbohydrates, and minerals that it actually needs. When these laxatives are taken most of the time the body hasn't had time to digest what it needs in order to survive and thrive.

Binge Eating Disorder

We've covered this type of eating extensively in

previous chapters. Binge eating stems mainly from eating to fill an emotional need rather than a physical (hunger) need. This eating disorder leaves us with many emotional scars, especially guilt and self-loathing.

Diet Pills

While diet pills in themselves aren't an eating disorder, becoming addicted to them can be dangerous. Whether it's weight loss pills, supplements or laxatives, they can all have long-term detrimental effects if they are used excessively.

There are literally hundreds of pills on the market that promise immediate results. This is one of the main reasons why there are so many diets available in the marketplace at the moment. It's a multi-billion-dollar industry that's growing daily and one that doesn't show signs of slowing down or stopping anytime soon.

Fasting or Intermittent Fasting

Many believe that this is a way to regulate the metabolism or recharge it, getting it kicked back into high gear once more with the promise of rebalancing any hormones that are out of whack. The only way to achieve this is by honoring your body and what it is telling you. Not by starving it from time to time. All that this achieves is getting the body to store more fat because it knows that there will come a time when it's not going to be fed.

Restrictive Dieting

Any diet that says that you should avoid certain foods or food groups is potentially harmful. If you were to visit any registered dietician, they would provide you with a proper breakdown of exactly what your body needs to survive. You'd be amazed that there are still fats included in these balanced diets because the body needs them to operate effectively. If a diet prevents you from eating anything—toss it out!

Skipping Meals

This is as close to fasting or intermittent fasting as you can get. Once again, if the body is feeling deprived of food, it's going to move into the 'store for later' phase. This is where fatty deposits begin to occur throughout the body so that it knows it has enough 'fuel' for the next time it's deprived. Starting to get the picture on why cutting back or cutting out completely actually leads to weight gain?

Steroids and/or Supplements

Part of this multi-billion-dollar industry. Many of these have not been tested accurately or they are used incorrectly. Because many of these are new to the industry they cannot always be accurately backed up by clinical trials. Pumping the body full of these chemicals is not a good thing. Even meal replacements such as protein shakes are never as effective as actually eating foods that contain protein. These supplements always contain other additives and ingredients that could have harmful side effects on the body if they are used over an extended period of time.

Unbalanced Food Intake

This is where certain food groups are removed from your food intake completely. An example of this would be cutting out carbohydrates, or protein from your diet. By restricting these foods from what should be a normal balanced diet, the body responds differently and begins to store fat. Even the body's metabolism is affected.

The recommendation when it comes to all these types of diets is to ignore all of them and aim for returning to a healthier, balanced lifestyle where you aren't restricted with what you can or cannot eat. It's learning to embrace food all over again and rediscover those foods that bring you joy. It's taking time to enjoy the food you're eating, learning how to savor it. When you reach this stage you will begin to embrace your body image for what it is and rather than feeling guilty or self-loathing, you will begin to replace these feelings with love, joy, and self-appreciation.

DEALING WITH DEPRESSION

Feelings of depression usually appear along with guilt attached to our eating habits. If we've 'broken' a diet by eating something on the 'bad food' list feelings of remorse can take over. These can begin with guilt as mentioned above but can quickly escalate to feelings of depression. This could lead to bouts of anxiety, panic attacks, self-isolation, low self-esteem and even self-hatred.

Depression can lead to complete withdrawal from society. Feeling too ashamed about our inability to remain strong enough to stick to a 'diet.'

This is no way for anyone to live. It's allowing your negative relationship with food to take over your life. By the time you reach this stage, you need to accept that you've moved past the point where you are in control. The 'diet' is now controlling you and you need help to get out of what seems to be a bottomless abyss of self-loathing, blame, and doubt in your ability to beat these feelings.

For some, you may have a strong support group to lean on who can easily coax you back from the edge and help you turn your current thoughts around. For others, counseling may be necessary. If you find yourself at this point, decide to change your Dieting Dilemma! Either turn to your support group and ask for help or pick up the phone and reach out to a professional counselor. This could be anyone from a Registered Dietician, to a psychologist or psychiatrist. Consider contacting your general practitioner in the first instance if you're experiencing constant low moods and feelings of depression.

Don't wait until you reach the point of no return. Know that there's always hope and help available out there.

HOW POSITIVE BODY IMAGE CAN ACTUALLY HELP YOU

We all understand the concept of the difference between something that's positive versus something that's negative. The same is true of how we feel towards our body image. When we can step back and appreciate our body for everything that it is and does for us on a daily basis, we may experience a positive shift in what we currently believe.

Understand and accept that we are all unique and have a distinct set of characteristics and personality traits that we can offer the world.

We have each been born to be unique and different and this is something to be celebrated. Imagine how boring the world would be if we all looked exactly the same, had the same measurements, wore the same shoe size, had the same eye color, hair color, skin tone, you get the idea. Can anyone say bland and boring?

Being different from each other is actually what sets us apart. It's why certain people are naturally drawn towards being more athletic than others. It's what separates the nerds from the jocks. We can't all be actors or supermodels either. Imagine the world without individuals that have made unique contributions or still continue to do so: Mahatma Gandhi, Nelson Mandela, Florence Nightingale, Madame Curie, Steve Jobs, Sir Richard Branson, Bill Gates, Oprah Winfrey, and the list can go on and on.

What about the valuable contributions that are yet to come as a result of the rising generation(s)? Are these going to be stymied or placed on hold because people don't like the way they look? Or because they are going to crack under the pressure that society places on them to look a certain way, dress a certain way, act a certain way?

There is too much negative emphasis being placed on body image. It needs to be replaced by encouraging individualism and celebrating and embracing diversity, rather than demanding 'cookie -compliance to body image.

Breaking the mold is going to be up to you and it's going to be the values you instill in your children. They are watching and learning from you daily and these lessons will be perpetuated and repeated in their own homes with their own children someday.

If you are currently restricting your family's eating habits because you're following some diet, you run the risk of harming future generations when it comes to their perceived relationship with certain foods.

It's better to teach your children the basics of what defines a healthy lifestyle, as well as intuitive eating habits, and encourage them to make their own decisions (obviously only once they are old enough).

We need to get back to the point in time where we become as little children—eat when you are hungry and once you've had enough, leave the rest. The mentality that most of us were raised with was as a result of the Depression (where you weren't certain where your next meal was coming from—so you ate what was in front of you). Today, we live in an environment where our cupboards, refrigerators, and freezers are full. We no longer need to be concerned about scarcity.

9

SURROUND YOURSELF WITH THE RIGHT ENVIRONMENT

"Make food choices that honor your health and taste buds while making you feel good. Remember that you don't have to eat a perfect diet to be healthy. You will not suddenly get a nutrient deficiency, or gain weight from one snack, one meal, or one day of eating. It's what you eat consistently over time that matters. Progress, not perfection, is what counts."

— EVELYN TRIBOLE

INVOLVING FAMILY

Getting the entire family on board with intuitive eating could present a challenge depending on how old your children are. Naturally, the earlier you are able to start teaching them about eating intuitively, the better it will be for all. Should your children be very young though, it's important that you don't overwhelm them with too many food choices per meal.

At the same time if you dislike certain foods, avoid

passing this aversion onto your children, even subconsciously. Allow them to make their own decisions regarding food preferences (as long as these don't only consist of fast foods). The emphasis here is on intuitively eating while choosing mainly those foods that are going to provide you with a balanced diet that is nutritional.

EAT TOGETHER

Starting to eat intuitively as a family is a perfect time to revive the age-old tradition of sitting down and enjoying your meals at a dinner table together as a family. Before televisions were invented, families would gather around the dinner table and communicate with each other face to face on all sorts of topics. There were no cell phones that demanded our constant attention or tv programs that we had just to watch. Dinners used to be a time of bonding and learning new things. It was also a time to discuss things that happened during the day. Parents actually knew what was happening in their children's lives and mealtimes were a fun part of the day.

Meals were consumed a lot more slowly as a result of each member of the family communicating with each other. This is what we need to be aiming for once more. Actually sitting down for meals. You could even consider making the dining area a 'cell-free/technology-free' zone for the duration of the meal. Make the meal and communication the focal point of the time that you spend together. This will allow you to channel your intuitive eating by enjoying your mealtime experience. As you take regular breaks while talking, before simply placing another helping of food into your mouth, think about where you are on the hunger—satisfaction scale? If you are satisfied, don't force yourself to clear your plate. Listen to your body, and honor both your hunger and your fullness.

When introducing intuitive eating to your family, although you may be the one responsible for what's dished up on everyone's plate, it should be up to them as to how much they eat.

Remember the toddler theory of only eating to the point where they're no longer hungry... this is what you're aiming for and this should be where you're aiming to get your family to as well. Let them decide when they've had enough.

If you're concerned about food being wasted, dish up smaller portions with the view that everybody can always have more if they are still hungry. In theory, the bigger the plate, the bigger the portion size that's served. If you know that you're definitely eating way too much food at the moment, look at replacing your current plates with ones that are smaller, and try to dish up proportionately to the plate. Be careful not to overload the plate as this may once again make you feel as though you must finish everything that's been served.

ALLOW CHILDREN TO DECIDE ON WHEN THEY ARE SATISFIED

Don't force-feed your children or insist that they eat everything in front of them. Part of the growing into the intuitive eating experience is discovering what foods you actually enjoy. Your family mealtimes should be happy times—that way you will experience and associate joy rather than pressure with food and mealtimes.

Don't pressurize family members to eat if they aren't hungry. For example, say that one of your children returned home from football practice and ate a fair size lunch around 4 pm: he's certainly not going to be in the mood to face another full-size meal at dinnertime at 6:30 pm. However, it will be worthwhile for his dinner to be placed in the refrigerator or microwave for when he actually is feeling hungry.

Remember the golden rule of intuitive eating—eat when you are hungry!

STOCK UP WITH HEALTHY SNACKS

Other ideas include ensuring that there are ready to nibble on snacks in healthy portion sizes stored in your refrigerator for easy access. You can also add these to your children's lunch boxes for school.

Healthy snacks could include anything from fresh fruits such as apples, pears, bananas, oranges, to cheese wedges or blocks of cheese cut into cubes. Boiled eggs are also a great option for a healthy snack as they can provide protein: the same goes for small amounts of meat or chicken.

As an idea for a more filling snack, for example for children who are active in sports at school, consider preparing a chicken salad that has added croutons and hard-boiled eggs.

Encourage your children to eat as many fruits and vegetables in their raw format, as it's in their raw form that they contain the most nutrients, making them the most beneficial.

STOCKING CUPBOARDS

Adding to the above, choose to stock your pantry with good, wholesome foods as much as possible. Ensure you make it as easy and quick as possible for you and your family to be able to whip up a healthy and tasty meal. For example, you can stock up on tins of chicken and/or fish that can be added to a fresh pasta salad quite quickly for a boost of protein. try to reduce the number of unhealthy snacks you stock on as they could be used as 'comfort food' when you're having a bad day. This would include all the usual suspects like cookies, chocolate bars, potato crisps, candy, and anything with high sugar content. Limit the amount of ice-cream available at any time in your freezer, and possibly replace it with frozen yogurt, or frozen fruits that can be blended into yummy and nutritional smoothies.

I'm not advocating that you don't have some treats to enjoy as a family: remember that the secret to intuitive eating is to have everything in moderation. Once you are used to feeding yourself with what you want, when you want, you will find that you experience fewer cravings for sweets and fast foods.

CHOOSE HEALTH OVER FAST FOOD

As a result of the fast-paced lifestyle most of us live, we've come to rely too heavily on the 'convenience' of fast food to replace a structured, well-balanced meal plan. This is where things begin to go sideways. It's easier for us to call for a pizza delivery or Chinese take-out, or stopping by Burger King on the way home from work, rather than taking the time to shop for food and prepare a proper home-cooked meal.

If you do a little research on the nutritional values of the most popular fast-food options, just one click away, you will find that most are actually extremely unhealthy as a food option.

If you really need to save time on food preparation, there are a number of alternatives that could be considered. Some of these include fresh fruit and vegetable outlets that sell fresh produce that's already been skinned and diced, literally ready to be added to the pot immediately with no preparation time at all. This goes for anything from frozen chopped mushrooms to crumbed onion rings. These may be slightly more expensive, but when you consider that you are paying for the fruit or vegetable by actual weight, without the skin and/or pips or seeds, you will realize that the costs are almost the same. Plus, there's something to be said for saving considerable amounts of time. If you are short on time and can afford the slightly more expensive option, they are worth it, as your time is precious.

These same food outlets sell meat and fish that's already filleted, prepared and ready to cook, making it easier than you could ever imagine to cook dinner from scratch. Almost anything you could imagine is available in a format that can be prepared fairly quickly with little to no fuss whatsoever. The benefit of going this route is that you can easily focus on big bouts of meal preparation to

EATING OUT (WHILE INTUITIVE EATING)

stock up your freezer or refrigerator with all the right food choices.

Once you are in tune with both your body and your hunger, eating out should be no different than eating at home. If you know the restaurant or food establishment and have an idea of their portion sizes, it becomes easier to order a smaller portion, or order your side dishes to share with others at the table. Consider ordering any additional sauces on the side, rather than having them serve them together with the meal. That way, you have control over how much sauce you decide to pour over your meal.

Remember that even when eating out, you don't need to finish everything on your plate. You can ask for it to be put in a container to take it home with you (seeing as you are paying for the entire meal, after all).

If you know that you are going to indulge yourself by having dessert after your meal, skip the starter, or vice versa. Because you are going to a restaurant, it doesn't mean that you MUST eat a 3-course meal. Sometimes the best meal to have in a restaurant is a buffet as this allows you to be in full control over how much and what you choose to eat.

When you aren't in control of the menu because you've been invited to attend an event such as a wedding or bar mitzvah and there is going to be a set menu—once again, you do not need to eat everything put in front of you! This mantra is beginning to sound like a war cry at this stage, because it actually is. Learn to stop eating when you are satisfied. Place your knife and fork down and allow your plate to be removed. Your body will thank you for it throughout the night and the following day.

If you are celebrating a special occasion, remember that having that slice of cake, or dessert is not going to suddenly make you obese. It's healthy to live with a balanced relationship with food. That means that you allow yourself those little luxuries from time to time. Remember that when the 'diet' mentality says that you need to cut something out of your diet—it almost automatically appears on the list of things that you will crave consistently. The quote at the beginning of this chapter says it so succinctly. You need to be able to experience joy together with your food, rather than opting for a life that is bland, tasteless, and uninteresting.

10

SEEKING HELP AND FINDING A COMMUNITY

"The greatness of a community is most accurately measured by the compassionate action of its members."

— *CORETTA SCOTT KING*

Recovery from any form of addiction takes time, compassion and usually requires the support of others to be fully effective. Recovering from compulsive dieting is exactly the same. There is no difference to the challenges faced by anyone who is so used to doing things in a certain way to having to physically unlearn them and learning something completely different.

WHERE TO GO FROM HERE?

In this final chapter, we are going to look at where you can find the help and assistance you need while you transition from life as a compulsive dieter to living as someone who learns the art of intuitive eating. Mentally it can be challenging and exhausting to figure out whether you're going about things the right way. How can you tell whether the voice inside your head is actually your intuition speaking to you, or it is just yourself? And, if so, is there a difference?

QUESTIONS AND ANSWERS

So many questions that need to be answered on this intuitive eating journey. These are only a few of them:

- How do I know what foods I really like?
- How can I pick up on when I am feeling hungry rather than being ravenous due to emotional turmoil?
- How will I know if my body is receiving enough nutrition?
- What do I do if I'm hungry again in the middle of the night?

Because most of our lives are so busy and we do so much on the go—it's easy to skip some of these hunger cues. For the first while, you are going to need to pay close attention to what your body is saying to you, as and when it happens. It's like learning to tune into a specific radio frequency where the station is coming through loud and clear and the static or background noise is blocked out.

The answers to most of these questions are all actually common sense—even though we are often told that this is not so common! The single most important thing to learn from your experiments with intuitive eating is to judge how you feel while you are eating. Once you are able to do that, everything else will fall into place, and you will be able to enjoy the taste and texture of the food that you are eating, maybe for the first time in your life since you were very little. You will be able to slow down to appreciate the explosion of flavor happening in your mouth ... something that you've probably forgotten about because you're so used to grabbing a quick bite and eating on the run.

SLOWING LIFE DOWN

Life demands more and more of our time and there doesn't seem to be any way of stopping the fast pace or slowing it down. While we may not be able to change modern society or the pace of our work life, there are a few things that are actually under our control. As discussed in an earlier chapter, for example, we can slow life down by sitting together at a table for meals with our family. It builds relationships with our loved ones and gives us the ideal opportunity for practicing listening to what our intuition is telling us regarding the relationship that we have with our food. This relationship can either create a positive experience, where we've been able to take our time and enjoy what is in front of us, or it can result in a haphazard experience as we grab something on the go, not paying any attention to the taste, texture, our hunger level or whether we are satisfied.

We should make a real effort to eliminate multitasking while eating. This way we can enhance our eating experience. Focusing on our food allows us to become fully present in the moment and allows us to reconnect with our food preferences, as well as being in control of what we are eating and when.

HOW CAN THERAPY HELP?

Therapy can come to our aid in various forms when it comes to intuitive eating. If you're a recovering obsessive-compulsive dieter or chronic dieter, breaking the calorie counting habits of the past can be extremely difficult to do. For many, the mere thought of shopping without scanning each and every label to check ingredients can be daunting. It will often take a complete shift in mindset to change the self-defeating dieting belief system.

In many instances, this requires professional intervention by those who are qualified to offer this counsel and advice. Depending on the severity of the belief system surrounding body image you have acquired over the years, this may need to be referred to specialists who are able to deal with mental issues.

We are each different and therefore have the capacity and ability to face challenges and overcome them in different ways. For some, transitioning from being a compulsive dieter to an intuitive eater could be fairly smooth sailing. They may be able to read the supporting statistics and case studies and be able to accept that no diets are beneficial in the long term. On the other hand, others may need to attend multiple sessions of therapy or counseling sessions with dieticians, psychologists or even psychiatrists. It would all depend on how their self-image, self-esteem, or body image has been damaged. Those suffering from severe depression cannot and will not just be able to 'snap out of it' magically. It's important to be realistic and understand that this will take time.

ONLINE COMMUNITIES

There are many online communities that are there to support you in your journey towards intuitive eating. These could be found via online search engines such as Google or Bing; they're also often listed on platforms like Facebook and LinkedIn and if you make use of geo-tagging, you could probably find an actual in-person community in your region. Joining one of these groups may be an ideal way to start off your intuitive eating journey. Other members could help you by sharing some of what they've experienced with you. They may be able to share some advice that you could either use or discard if it's not really applicable to you. The upside of being able to communicate with those who have gone through it before you is that they are able to share some of the mistakes that they may have made in the past. This can help you avoid repeating these same mistakes yourself. Additionally, a community can offer a welcome reminder that you're not alone in this journey of self-acceptance and self-discovery. You may even make some new, non-dieting friends!

APPOINT A FRIEND

Share what you are doing with a close friend. Ask them to help you by holding you accountable. It needs to be someone that you can trust and that is strong enough to stand up to you and let you know when you're slipping, or out of line. Ways that they can hold you accountable is by setting specific goals with them. The journals that we've discussed throughout this book could be shared with them so they can monitor how you're doing. You could also schedule regular times to get together to discuss your progress. Don't procrastinate these meetings. Set them weekly for the first while, until you are feeling more confident and comfortable.

Once you've got the handle on it and you are comfortable with being able to hear your intuition telling you when you're hungry and when you've had enough, you can begin setting your meetings further apart. As much as possible, meet up in person. It's not as easy to hide what you're really experiencing when you're face to face.

ADDITIONAL RESOURCES

Since Evelyn Tribole and Elyse Resch first wrote *Intuitive Eating* in 1995, followers of this way of eating and living have popped up all over the world. Support groups are available, training is available, and research is ongoing even though it's been 25 years since this work was originally published. This should provide anyone wanting to kick the dieting habit for good a clear incentive that they won't be faced with doing it alone. Those who have managed to master it will be there right alongside you each step of the way.

AFTERWORD

Kicking the Diet Mindset has provided you with all the tools and information that you should ever need to never again be sucked into being duped into another diet fad, fashion, formula, or trends that makes promises it cannot keep. Instead of promising you miraculous weight loss overnight (the Nirvana of all things diet-related), intuitive eating allows you to completely change the way you think about food.

BAN THE BILLBOARDS

Intuitive eating is about taking control back and listening to your inner voice when it comes to eating rather than listening to what society is telling you instead. Society will always be in your face brandishing billboards, geo-tagging the websites you visit and spewing out images of the perfect look, the perfect image, the perfect body, shape, size, etc. Realize that all of these are just advertising gimmicks and tactics to get you to buy their products (in many instances, for you, this may be diet-related). Don't let them get into your head. Remember how many diets you've already tried and failed. That's been one of your main reasons for buying this book: you have been in search of a better way, a healthier way of doing things.

FOLLOWING THE FAMOUS

Following the lives of celebrities closely on Facebook, Instagram or Twitter can trigger strong emotions of negative body image or self-loathing because you don't look like them. What all of these advertising agencies, film companies and modeling agencies don't tell you is how much makeup is being applied, how much photoshopping takes place before things go to print or hit the marketplace. The pressure of conforming to the stereotypes that society demands we blindly accept as 'the norm', or the world requires, is too much to handle for most of us.

The secret to eliminating most of the pressure from how all of these images that you're surrounded with constantly is to get rid of as many of them as possible. It's learning to discover exactly who you are from the inside out—rather than from the outside in. The saying "beauty is only skin deep," by Sir Thomas Overbury (1613) is something that we should embrace and even write down and place in a prominent place in your home. This will remind you not to become preoccupied with your physical appearance to the point where it's leaving you miserable and depressed.

The solution to this problem is a simple one: hit the "unfollow" or "unlike" button on all of these accounts and begin looking for websites, forums, online communities and even celebrities that boost your self-image and your self-confidence. Sign up for these instead. There are loads of positive influencers for good out there who aren't going to make you empty promises at a high cost. Find the right accounts to follow and embrace the freedom that comes from finally understanding that looking 'perfect' isn't actually that important at all!

LEARN TO LOVE YOURSELF

Learning to love yourself as you are is one of the main aims of intuitive eating. It's retraining yourself to rediscover or form a new relationship with the food that you eat. Intuitive eating gives you back freedom from stressing about overindulging or binge eating. It skips past the guilt trip that potentially leads to anxiety and depression, which leads to further binge eating of comfort food ... and so the cycle continues.

Loving yourself promotes self-acceptance as you are right now, at this moment. It's not asking you to prove anything to anyone. You don't need to be a size 2 to be invited to this party of positive emotions. You can simply revert to reading through the list that you made in your journal about all the good things your body can do for you right now. As you become stronger, you will find that your lists will become even longer, allowing you to celebrate even more positive attributes. Celebrate each aspect of your body as it is right at this moment—recognizing what it's capable of and even what it can't do, and being at peace with that.

Come to terms with your body and learn to be okay with it. For many, this process is more like a journey that needs to be explored and discovered over time. Intuitive eating involves no magic lotions, potions, pills, or programs that are going to make you instantly lose weight that's making you feel bad about yourself. Instead, it breaks the chains of conventional diets that require calorie counting, weighing out portions or calculating how many calories you've managed to burn during the day in order to plan your evening meal. Intuitive eating sets you free from all of this stress and anxiety by going back to your roots, maybe for the first time in your life from when you were a toddler and your mother allowed you to eat whatever you wanted, leaving things on your plate and making your own decisions when it came to food. This is the point that you're trying to get back to.

PUT YOUR BODY BACK IN CHARGE

Intuitive eating puts your body back in the driving seat by teaching you to listen to when your body tells you you're hungry, rather than eating for the sake of eating. By listening to the same promptings that will let you know that you've had sufficient food to fuel your body, you'll begin to take back the control that's defined your relationship with food for most of your life. Allow yourself to make the decisions on what types of foods you want to eat. Choose those that you most enjoy and that make you feel happy. There's nothing worse than feeling that you have to drink only tomato and celery juice for a month in an attempt to shed a few pounds (not that intuitive eating is about losing weight).

AFTERWORD

LICENSE TO CHOOSE

Intuitive eating is not a license to go out there and binge-eat anything and everything, although this may be a learning curve that you need to go through to discover that there are consequences for not listening to when the body tells you it's full. Having to experience bloating and other side effects of overeating could allow you to begin to recognize what happens when you don't stop.

Intuitive eating is not a diet, it has not and never will be flaunted and promoted as a diet—not even going back to its original introduction in 1995 was it promoted as such. It's always been regarded as a way of finally ending the intimate war between yourself and food.

FORGIVING YOURSELF

Intuitive eating is about forgiving yourself for the way you look now. You may have been a victim of the dieting merry-go-round, on again and off again. Each time gaining slightly more weight than the time before. It's time to stop blaming your current weight issues on anything other than poor food relationships or choices. With intuitive eating, the buck needs to stop with you. You need to take full responsibility and ownership of your health, your body, and the food that you're choosing to put into your body.

Your old eating habits are now in the past. Clean the slate and make a decision to move on. Don't waste any valuable time by looking back at failed dieting attempts. If you begin this journey with intuitive eating, you need to be prepared to forgive yourself of all past choices and decisions and learn to let go.

CHOOSE HEALTH AND VITALITY

Intuitive eating is taking a holistic view of your health and vitality, especially when it relates to food. Accept and appreciate that you're not going to get the whole intuitive eating thing down immediately. It's going to be a process. It's going to be a journey. If you choose to share it with your family, friends, or other loved ones, it becomes more bearable because they will hold you accountable. Having to check in with someone to discuss how it's going makes it more difficult to return to old ways.

Being healthier through making better food choices will always influence and impact other areas of your life. It's not about losing weight, but rather about choosing a lifestyle that's going to lead to improved health and happiness.

OLD HABITS DIE HARD

Be patient with yourself when you catch yourself still counting calories in a store or reading food labels. Remind yourself that you no longer need to do that. Allow yourself the freedom to enjoy treats occasionally. Remember that one slice of cake or pizza is not going to destroy your lifestyle. Remind yourself over and over again that intuitive eating is a lifestyle rather than a diet. Give yourself the time that you need to make the changes in your eating patterns. Although this may be difficult to do at first, as you practice listening and watching for the hunger cues that your body provides you with, you will realize when you need to eat and when to set your knife and fork down.

ENJOY YOUR MEALS

Take your time over meals, reintroduce old traditions of eating at a dinner table once more. Celebrate the food that's in front of you, savoring it by eating more slowly than you normally would if you were multi-tasking. If you're in the workplace, make a point of not eating at your desk while you're working. Instead, get up and eat your meal in a canteen, on a park bench or somewhere away from the office.

Allowing yourself to be distracted while eating could often allow for overeating to occur. Because your focus is divided between your meal and your work, your phone, or the tv, it becomes impossible to hear the body's cues that are telling you that you have had enough.

Chew your food thoroughly and take smaller bite sizes versus shoveling everything down in a matter of seconds. Not only will this give you time to savor the food in front of you, but you'll enjoy the meal more. Greater appreciation for the taste of the food leads to feeling satisfied. This is the point where you need to set your knife and fork down.

ALLOW YOU TO BE YOU

The most important key to intuitive eating is to allow yourself to be who you truly are. It's falling in love with yourself and accepting your body the way that it is right

AFTERWORD

now. While we've spoken about keeping journals for your food journey and activities, you could either add to it, or you can do this by beginning and keeping a new journal of all the things you're grateful for that your body can do, as it is—right now!

It's replacing feelings of self-loathing with feelings of self-care and learning to be kinder and gentler towards yourself. Self-love is centered on accepting that we are all unique and have something to contribute to the world. Discovering exactly what this is may take time, effort, and some deep soul-searching. It's getting to know exactly who you are and loving yourself for it. In a world that wants you to think you're not enough (so that people can sell you things), self-love is a revolutionary act. Be brave!

MOVING FORWARD

Your personal journey towards self-discovery through intuitive eating is just one step away. All that it needs from you is a desire to begin... Remember that there are people out there who have walked this path before you. There are support groups and online communities just waiting for you to reach out and join them.

All that it's going to take on your part is a willingness to walk away from the dieting mentality forever and look at discovering exactly who you are. You are strong enough—you've got this!

REFERENCES

(2017). Exercise 'keeps the mind sharp' in over-50s, study finds. – BBC News. https://www.bbc.com/news/health-39693462

10 Principles of Intuitive Eating. (n.d.). https://www.intuitiveeating.org/10-principles-of-intuitive-eating/

10 Steps to Positive Body Image. (n.d.). https://www.nationaleatingdisorders.org/learn/general-information/ten-steps

Barghouty, L. (2020). What Intuitive Eating Can & Can't Do, According To Experts. https://www.bustle.com/p/what-intuitive-eating-can-cant-do-according-to-experts-21814401

Barraclough, E. L., Hay-Smith, E. J. C., Boucher, S. E., Tylka, T. L., Howarth, C. C., (2019). Learning to eat intuitively: A qualitative exploration of the experience of mid-age women. https://www.ncbi.nlm.nih.gov/pmc/articles/PMC6360478

Barker, M. (2019). Intuitive eating: a 'diet' that actually makes sense. https://theconversation.com/intuitive-eating-a-diet-that-actually-makes-sense-112800

Bendsen, N. T., et al. (2013). Is Beer Consumption Related to Measures of Abdominal and General Obesity? A Systematic Review and Meta-Analysis - PubMed. https://pubmed.ncbi.nlm.nih.gov/23356635/

Benito-Corchon, S., Bes-Rastollo, M. (2014). Glycemic load, glycemic index, bread and incidence of overweight/obesity in a Mediterranean cohort: the SUN project. BMC Public Health. doi:10.1186/1471-2458-14-1091

Benshosan, A. (2018). The Reason Most Americans Diet Isn't Weight Loss—It's This. https://www.eatthis.com/reason-people-go-diet/

Body Image. (n.d.). https://www.nationaleatingdisorders.org/body-image-0

Brazier, Y. (2017). Body image: What is it and how can I improve it? https://www.medicalnewstoday.com/articles/249190

Bruce, L. J., Ricciardelli, L. A. (2016). A systematic review of the psychosocial correlates of intuitive eating among adult women. https://www.sciencedirect.com/science/article/abs/pii/S0195666315300635

Cash, T. F., Smolak, L. (2011). Body Image, Second Edition: A Handbook of Science, Practice, and Prevention. New York: Guilford Press.

Dillon, J. D. (n.d.). The Love Food Podcast. https://podcasts.apple.com/us/podcast/the-love-food-podcast/id1076673018

Disordered Eating & Dieting. (n.d.). https://www.nedc.com.au/eating-disorders/eating-disorders-explained/disordered-eating-and-dieting/

Dodier, S. (2019). Intuitive Eating Made Simple: A Step-by-Step Guide. https://thriveglobal.com/stories/intuitive-eating-made-simple-a-step-by-step-guide/

Downs, M. (n.d.). Why Do We Keep Falling for Fad Diets? https://www.webmd.com/diet/features/why-do-we-keep-falling-for-fad-diets

Flores, A. (2018). What Does Intuitive Eating Mean? https://www.nationaleatingdisorders.org/blog/what-does-intuitive-eating-mean

Frey, M. (2019). How to Start a Workout Routine If You're Overweight. https://www.verywellfit.com/best-workouts-if-youre-overweight-3495993

Gavin, M. L. (n.d.). The Deal With Diets (for Teens) – Nemours KidsHealth. https://kidshealth.org/en/teens/dieting.html

Gingell, S. (2018). How Your Mental Health Reaps the Benefits of Exercise: New research shows why physical exercise is essential to mental health. https://www.psychologytoday.com/za/blog/what-works-and-why/201803/how-your-mental-health-reaps-the-benefits-exercise

Harrison, C. (n.d.) Podcast - Christy Harrison - Intuitive Eating Dietician, Anti-Diet Author, & Health at Every Size Advocate - Food Psych Programs. https://christyharrison.com/foodpsych

Hartley, R. (2015). Three Exercises for Newbie Intuitive Eaters. https://www.rachaelhartleynutrition.com/blog/2015/06/exercises-for-new-intuitive-eaters

Heart Matters Magazine. 10 Principles of intuitive eating. (n.d.). https://www.bhf.org.uk/informationsupport/heart-matters-magazine/nutrition/weight/intuitive-eating/10-principles-of-intuitive-eating

Hunt, T. (2019). Intuitive Eating Sounds Great, But What If I Still Want To Lose Weight? https://tailored-coachingmethod.com/intuitive-eating/

Imma Eat That. (n.d.). https://immaeatthat.com/

Intuitive Eating Quotes by Evelyn Tribole. (n.d.) https://www.goodreads.com/work/quotes/228458-intuitive-eating-a-revolutionary-program-that-works

Jennings, K. (2019). A Quick Guide to Intuitive Eating. https://www.healthline.com/nutrition/quick-guide-intuitive-eating

John Hopkins Medicine. (n.d.). Exercising for Better Sleep https://www.hopkinsmedicine.org/health/wellness-and-prevention/exercising-for-better-sleep

Johnson, B. (2012). Mind - Body - Nutrition: Nutritional psychologist Marc David explains why our mental and emotional responses to food matter far more than we realize. https://experiencelife.com/article/mind-body-nutrition/

Jones, J. (2019). So You Want to Try Intuitive Eating, but If You're Being Honest, You Still Want to Watch Your Weight. What to Do? https://www.self.com/story/intuitive-eating-and-weight-loss

Karges, C. (n.d.). Intuitive Eating Principles as a Family. https://www.eatingdisorderhope.com/blog/learning-intuitive-eating-principles-as-a-family

Landsverk, G. (2020). 'Intuitive eating' is on the rise, and experts say it's because people are fed up with diet culture. https://www.insider.com/what-is-intuitive-eating-does-it-work-2020-1

Leal, D. (2020). Improve Your Health With Intuitive Eating: Say "No" to Diets and "Yes" to a Healthy Relationship With Food. https://www.verywellfit.com/overview-of-intuitive-eating-4178361

London, J. (2019). What Is Intuitive Eating? How to Eat Better Without Dieting, According to Nutritionists: Forget calorie counting and food restricting—this philosophy is all about listening to your body. https://www.goodhousekeeping.com/health/diet-nutrition/a26324845/intuitive-eating/

Mandl, E. (2019). Binge Eating Disorder: Symptoms, Causes, and Asking for Help. https://www.healthline.com/nutrition/binge-eating-disorder

Muhlheim, L. (2020). How Can Intuitive Eating Help My Eating Disorder? https://www.verywellmind.com/intuitive-eating-can-help-disordered-eating-4796957

Nutrition Matters Podcast | Positive Nutrition. (n.d.). https://www.positive-nutrition.com/podcast

Positive Body Image. (n.d.). https://www.skillsyouneed.com/ps/positive-body-image.html

Quotes About The Power of Community. (n.d.). https://www.ellevatenetwork.com/articles/8538-quotes-about-the-power-of-community

Rollin, J. (2015). 3 Reasons You Should Never Go on a Diet: Research shows a surprising percentage of us simply can't keep it off long-term. https://www.psychologytoday.com/us/blog/mindful-musings/201510/3-reasons-you-should-never-go-diet

Rumsey, A. (2017). How to Get Started with Intuitive Eating. https://alissarumsey.com/intuitive-eating/how-to-start-intuitive-eating/

Rumsey, A. (2017). Ask Yourself This Before (and

Rumsey, A. (2018). Listen to Your Body Using the Hunger Fullness Scale – What to Eat (and When You Should Stop After) You Eat. https://alissarumsey.com/nutrition/hunger-fullness-scale/

Rumsey, A. (2019). How to Practice Intuitive Movement. https://alissarumsey.com/fitness/intuitive-exercise-tips/

Rumsey, A. (2019). What is Intuitive Eating? https://www.alissarumsey.com/intuitive-eating/what-is-intuitive-eating/

Sauer, M., Olsen, N. (2018). 7 Things I Learned During My First Week of Intuitive Eating. https://www.healthline.com/health/my-first-week-of-intuitive-eating

Schaefer, J. T., Magnuson, A. B. (2014). A Review of Interventions that Promote Eating by Internal Cues | Science Direct https://www.sciencedirect.com/science/article/abs/pii/S2212267213018960

Stenovec, L. (n.d.). The Embodied & Well mom show. https://www.intuitiveeatingmoms.com/podcast-2/

The Foodie Dietitian Blog by Kara Lydon, RD | Kara Lydon (n.d.). https://karalydon.com/blog

The Phrase Finder: The meaning and origin of the expression: Beauty is only skin deep. (n.d.). https://www.phrases.org.uk/meanings/59200.html

The Real Life RD, (n.d.). https://www.thereallife-rd.com

Timmons, J., Pletcher, P. (2016). How Sedentary Obese People Can Ease Into Regular Exercise. https://www.healthline.com/health/fitness-exercise/exercise-for-obese-people

To thine own self be true – eNotes Shakespeare Quotes. (n.d.). https://www.enotes.com/shakespeare-quotes/thine-own-self-true

Tribole, E. (n.d.). Intuitive Eating Resources.

https://www.evelyntribole.com/resources/intuitive-eating-resources/

Van Dyke, N., Drinkwater, E. J., (2014). Relationships between intuitive eating and health indicators: literature review. – PubMed. https://www.ncbi.nlm.nih.gov/pubmed/23962472

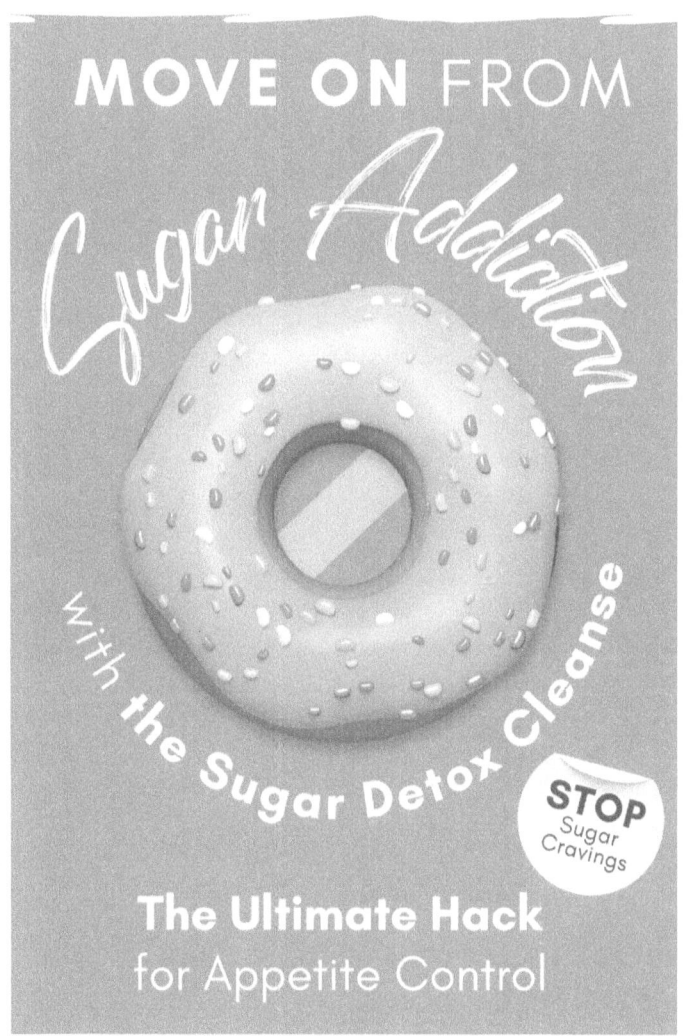

INTRODUCTION

"Success is the sum of small efforts—repeated day-in and day-out." —Robert Collier

Sugar is everywhere in our diets. It is present in everything from lattes at breakfast to brownies for dessert, and it is often included in every meal in between. It is easy to identify sugar when it is added to sweet treats, but it often flies under the radar and enters our diets unnoticed. Sugar hides in foods we generally perceive as healthy; the saying "an apple a day keeps the doctor away" might be true if it wasn't for the high amounts of naturally occurring sugar found in most varieties of apples. People who believe they are eating healthy may actually be consuming a great deal of sugar, and because of this, they do not understand why they struggle to maintain a healthy weight or keep potential health complications at bay.

Sugar's ability to masquerade in such a variety of forms is what makes it a health hazard to us. Despite the dangers, most people consume far too much sugar in their daily diet. Studies have found that an average American diet contains "22 to 30 teaspoons" of sugar a day, which is "considerably more than the recommended maximum of 6 teaspoons" (Santos-Longhurst, 2018, para. 4). But why is it that we are so prone to overindulgence when it comes to sweet things? A lack of knowledge about the real dangers sugar poses to our health, combined with the addictive nature of sugar, results in unhealthy sugar consumption habits.

Eating sugar is a vicious cycle. We often crave sugar when we are bored, stressed, or just looking for a treat to liven up our day. Eating a cookie seems like a harmless enough vice to engage in, and we get the added benefit of boosting our energy levels, however temporary that boost may be. However, after the energy boost comes the inevitable crash, and a sugar crash is especially severe. In a crash we often end up looking for more snacks, which leads us back to eating more sugar. Before long, we have become entirely dependent on sugar.

Sugar may be compelling for many of us, but can it really be called an addiction? Though cakes and cookies seem more benign than alcohol or cigarettes, they are actually just as addictive, and the term "sugar addiction" is no exaggeration. Sugar causes a dopamine spike in our brains, which temporarily boosts our moods. For people who struggle with frequent low moods and related health conditions like high stress levels and depression, this minor mood lift becomes a compulsion, and sugar becomes the main way low moods are managed. In fact, "some studies have suggested sugar is as addictive as cocaine," (Murray, 2020, para. 2). Once an addiction begins, we become more resistant to our dopamine spikes, which means we must consume more sugar to

INTRODUCTION

achieve the same feelings. We take larger and larger "hits" of sugar until the majority of our diet contains sugar in some form—all without realizing just how dependent we have become. This leads to higher sugar consumption and a greater risk of developing dangerous health conditions.

Additionally, like many other addictions, sugar negatively impacts your health while simultaneously encouraging you to consume more and more of a dangerous substance. An addiction to sugar is a serious health concern that many people struggle with throughout their lives. High sugar levels in your body make health problems such as diabetes, high blood pressure, inflammation, and heart disease more likely to occur.

Because our bodies have become so used to our high sugar diets, it is often hard to quit sugar. It is present in a wide range of food and drinks, from fruits to alcohol to baked goods, and everything in between. We tend to naturally seek out sweet things, and trying to lower our sugar consumption makes us more likely to crave the very thing we are attempting to quit. If you attempt to cut sugar out of your diet, you may even experience symptoms of withdrawal, just as you would if you tried to stop smoking. These symptoms can include more intense cravings, nausea, mood swings, and fluctuating energy levels.

Despite these difficulties, it is incredibly important to replace a diet high in sweets with one that is good for your body and your mind. Ending your sugar addiction is one of the best things you can do for yourself. Your health depends on your ability to moderate the presence of sugar in your diet.

INTRODUCTION

THE IMPORTANCE OF KICKING YOUR SUGAR HABIT

Sugar is much more dangerous than its sweet taste implies. While sugar tastes great and our bodies may crave it, the excessive sugar levels in most Americans' diets does them no favors. Sugar is one of the leading causes of obesity. If you're having trouble managing your weight, you should review just how much sugar you're really eating. It also commonly leads to inflammation and high blood pressure. Together, these conditions can drastically increase the likelihood of more serious health problems. They cause your cardiovascular system to struggle to keep up with your body's needs, which puts strain on your heart and your arteries. If left unchecked, this can develop into heart disease, which can be a life-threatening condition.

Kicking a sugar habit is hard, but with the right information and the right plan, you can increase your chances of successfully lowering the amount of sugar in your diet. You do not have to be controlled by your cravings any longer. Your sugar addiction will be a thing of the past. With the help of this book and the steps outlined in the sugar detox cleanse, you can improve your meal habits, routinely make healthier choices, and begin the journey towards a healthier life.

I know firsthand the dangers of sugar, which is why I am so committed to providing you with the best possible plan for ending your sugar addiction. Food was a coping mechanism for me in my youth. I used sugary snacks as an outlet for my struggles in my personal life, and as a result, I struggled with obesity and developed type 2

INTRODUCTION

diabetes at just 35 years old. I knew I had to make a change, and I needed to make one that would last, or my health would be in serious danger. By learning healthier coping mechanisms and developing better nutrition habits, I lost over 200 pounds in three years. I also developed healthy habits that have stuck with me every year since. I want to show you how to make changes in your diet, especially in regards to sugar, that will support the development of a more positive relationship with food.

It is time to stop letting sugar control you. Whether you are trying to prevent future health issues or you need to make changes to your diet to manage health conditions that have already developed, the sugar detox cleanse can help you beat your not-so-sweet addiction. This book will provide you with a better understanding of why sugar is such a difficult addiction to quit, as well as steps anyone can use to remove excessive sugar from your diet. By moving on from your sugar addiction, you can improve your relationship with food as a whole and support a healthier lifestyle.

1

THE EMOTIONAL ASPECTS OF SUGAR ADDICTION

WHY GIVING UP THE SWEETS IS SO HARD

Sugar is notoriously hard to quit. Many people who try to eat less sugar find themselves falling back into old habits, regardless of how many reasons there are to minimize its presence in our diets. This may even be something you have attempted previously before with little success. You may be tempted to chalk it up to just how many foods we eat every day that contain sugar—it is present in everything from fruit, to candy, to bread and pasta, which can make it hard to avoid. However, this doesn't fully account for the power of sugar's temptation and the frequency of sugar cravings when compared to many other types of food. After all, people quit eating certain foods all the time, even those which make up a great deal of a standard diet. People who develop gluten intolerance or celiac disease cut out bread and find replacements to make all their meals gluten-free. Becoming vegan or vegetarian means removing many meat products from your meal plans. You could probably stop eating some less popular foods like Brussels sprouts and chard without too much difficulty. What is it about sugar that makes it so difficult to cut out of your diet?

Sugar's power over us is a result of its connection to our emotions. Unlike many foods, our consumption of sugar has a direct impact on our brain chemistry. Rather than just filling us up, sugar makes us feel happier. It releases dopamine in our brains, and when we get that dopamine rush we become compelled to seek it out more and more often. We are constantly seeking out the source of momentary happiness that sugar provides, and the longer we spend chasing our "sugar high," the more sugar we must consume to get the same result. Think of how you consumed candy as a kid. It is very likely that back then, only a piece or two of chocolate was enough to send you into a sugar rush. Your brain responded much more strongly to the presence of sugar because it was a minimal part of your diet. Now, however, the same amount of sugar isn't likely to have you bouncing off the walls; it may not have an effect on your mood at all. Instead we must eat much more sugar to get the same results, which only makes it harder to end our sugar addictions. The more sugar we eat, the more change we would need to make to our eating habits to end our dependence on sugar.

Addiction to sugar is especially strong for those struggling with mental health and mood issues, and it is especially hard to quit as a result. You might be unknowingly using sugar as a way to cope with negative emotions. Many people who have experienced traumatic events or who suffer from depression and anxiety reach for sweet snacks when they are reminded of a negative event. Sugar makes us feel happier, and it can even balance us out when we enter an emotionally volatile state. The boost from sugar makes it easier to bring your mood back up, but it also means that you are managing your mood in a dangerous way. Continued use of sugar to regulate your emotions can lead to many health problems as sugar consumption gets out of hand.

Sugar dependency is comparable to an eating disorder, and it is often a component of stress eating and binge eating. Food serves as a way to calm your nerves, improve your mood, and manage other unfavorable factors in your life. You may feel a compulsion to eat when you are having trouble handling a recent development and your emotional state suffers. However, overindulging and eating the wrong things leads to health scares, especially when what you are eating has a high sugar content. It is harder and harder to end this behavior because eating sugar makes you feel good, while restricting your cravings gives you no such immediate gratification. While you may feel better in the long run if you end these behaviors, managing them in the short-term can leave you feeling unmotivated, lacking energy, and flip-flopping between emotional extremes.

This is the harmful and potentially even deadly trap of sugar. Under the sweet veneer lies a dangerous substance that is highly addictive because it preys on emotional vulnerability. It is so easy to become addicted to sugar because it seems like a relatively harmless addiction compared to others, but in reality the many hidden dangers and the cycle of dependence it creates can keep you trying to kick your sugar habit for years if you don't have the right strategy.

SIGNS YOU'RE ADDICTED TO SUGAR

You might eat sugar fairly regularly, but is the situation really so out of control? How do you know if you're addicted to sugar? Some people consume sugary foods as an occasional treat without feeling a strong desire to continue eating it, while others develop a real addiction. Of course, everything is fine in moderation, but the key defining trait of a sugar addiction is that moderation becomes impossible. You may be addicted to sugar if you experience any of the following behaviors and thought patterns.

You Crave Sugary Snacks Constantly

In one way or another, sugar is always on your mind. In much the same way as smokers are often thinking about their next cigarette, you are near-constantly thinking about the next time you can have sugar. This may be a craving for something sweet in general, or it may be a desire for a particular sugary comfort food that you have come to associate with improving your mood. Whatever shape your personal sugar craving takes, the only time it is not occupying your thoughts is when you are currently indulging in it.

Though sugar cravings may be persistent, this doesn't mean that they are always recognizable. Some cravings may lurk under the surface, and only when you begin to feel bored or snackish do you immediately default to looking for something sweet. You can focus on other, more important things in the meantime, but that desire for sugar sits at the back of your mind and strikes at its first opportunity.

Constant cravings can lead to irregular eating habits.

Ideally, you should be eating your meals around the same time each day. Snacking heavily in between, or taking meals at odd hours as a result of powerful cravings, completely throws off your daily meal schedule. You may find yourself having more late-night snacks, or waiting to eat dinner until very late because you spent the day snacking. Without regular meal times, you will find yourself feeling hungry nearly all the time, which can worsen the compulsion to overeat.

Bad Moods Make Your Cravings Worse

Because sugar has such a strong impact on your emotional state, you begin to associate eating sugar with feeling happier. This causes you to seek a solution for a bad mood in the form of sugar. When your mood dips and you start to feel agitated, you get a powerful desire to eat something sweet. This may be a conscious thought, or you may find yourself unconsciously snacking or reaching for a sugary drink. The compulsion to use sugar to handle a bad mood furthers your dependency on sugar, worsening the addiction. Your brain correlates feeling good with eating sugar and you start seeking it out to remedy even minor mood dips. When you are denied sugar, your mood falls even further, leading to more frequent bouts of irritability.

Though sugar provides a temporary mood and energy boost, it is not long-lasting, and it does little to deal with the reasons behind your bad mood. It's like slapping a bandage over the problem without dealing with the actual injury. You may feel a bit better in the moment, but whatever caused that bad mood will not be fixed. Negative thoughts that are a product of mental health issues or trauma will continue to persist without being adequately addressed. By quelling the thoughts with sugar, you simultaneously increase their frequency and lower the likelihood of seeking out better coping strategies for these mood swings.

You Eat Even When You Are Not Hungry

When you are addicted to sugar, you start seeking out sugar as often as possible. This means that you will often snack between meals. If you don't have much to do, you might head for the fridge or pantry and take a look around. Eventually, you start to eat whenever you are bored or looking for a small boost, which means you might be snacking near-constantly throughout the day.

You may be driven to eat, especially sugary foods, because you aren't able to find an outlet for certain issues. Low energy and boredom are common triggers, both of which can be solved in different ways. When you choose to eat instead of finding another, healthier method for revitalizing yourself, you encourage your own reliance on sugar.

You Frequently Engage in Overeating

As mentioned above, eating more often and seeking out food when you aren't hungry is a gateway to overeating. Overeating is very difficult to stop once you start. This is because you are essentially training your stomach to accept and crave more food than you would otherwise need. When you overeat, your stomach expands to make room for the food; this is why you may feel bloated, distended, and uncomfortable when you eat too much in one sitting. When binge eating occurs on a regular basis, you increase the capacity of your stomach gradually over time. This means you are hungry more often and you must eat more to satisfy your hunger. It is very hard to lose weight and manage your eating habits at this point because you can no longer have smaller meals and feel satisfied. This only leads to more overeating, starting the cycle anew.

After overeating, you may feel very sluggish as your body attempts to digest everything. This is especially true of high-carb meals, and as you may know, carbs are just more complex forms of sugars that are broken back down into simple sugar molecules in your body. It takes energy to break these molecules down, which is why you might feel so tired after a big bowl of pasta. Even though sugars provide your body with energy, that energy is often short-lived and the crash is typically worse than the initial energy boost. Additionally, many carbs contain tryptophan, which is an amino acid that can cause you to feel drowsy. Eating sugar traps you in a cycle of overeating, energy fluctuations, and often guilt as a result of your inability to control your eating habits.

You Experience Sugar-Related Health Problems

Sugar is a perfect example of how having "too much of a good thing" can be very harmful. While a little sugar in moderation is fine, eating too much sugar on a regular basis increases your likelihood of developing various health problems. One of the most notable health concerns related to sugar is the tendency for spikes and dips in your blood sugar. An instability in your blood sugar can make you tired more often, and it can put you in a bad mood more frequently, which just causes you to seek out sugar once again. The hormone responsible for managing your blood sugar level in your body is called insulin. When functioning normally, insulin removes and stores excess energy in the form of glucose, or sugar, from your bloodstream and moves it into your cells. However, when we eat excessive amounts of sugar, the insulin receptors in your cells start ignoring the presence of this hormone. This is a condition known as insulin resistance. It is a precursor to many more troubling health conditions that occur because your body can no longer process the sugar you eat. These health conditions include strokes, heart disease, and type two diabetes.

Type two diabetes is a particularly concerning health condition that can affect your life for years to come. It develops as a direct result of insulin resistance. Your body responds to your cells' inability to use insulin by producing even more insulin in your pancreas. The role insulin is meant to fulfill is not getting completed, so your body doesn't know how else to react other than to redouble its efforts. Eventually, your pancreas cells get worn out from the overproduction and can't keep pace, which means your insulin levels start to sharply drop. This results in a rise in your blood sugar that ultimately develops into type two diabetes when not appropriately addressed (Harrar, 2019, para. 4). By the time you are diagnosed with diabetes, insulin resistance has been occurring for a long time. It is merely the product of months or years of sugar addiction.

Another health condition that may develop as a result of too much sugar in your diet is metabolic syndrome. This is not just one health problem, but instead it represents a large group of related health issues, many of which have very few symptoms and can linger under the surface until more severe conditions develop. Metabolic syndrome includes high blood sugar, high blood pressure, high cholesterol, and excess body fat, especially around the waist area. These smaller problems build to form a much more dangerous whole. They can lead to grave health issues that threaten your ability to lead a healthy and happy life.

A LACK of Sugar Brings Bad Moods

When our emotions are tied to our sugar consumption, it is only natural that a lack of sugar will bring on bad moods more frequently. If you are addicted to sugar, you will become irritable if you go too long without any sugar or if you don't have enough sugar in a period of time. You may find yourself seeking it out to deal with these moods, and when you do get some sugar, you will associate the alleviation of your bad mood with the sugary snack or drink.

Because sugar is an addiction, attempting to abruptly cut it out of your diet can highlight just how dependent on it you have become. Many people have even said that trying to quit sugar led them to experience symptoms that were similar to withdrawal. You may feel more powerful cravings, more frequent mood swings, and physical malaise all because your body is not getting the amount of sugar it is used to.

SUGAR DETOX

An addiction to sugar is more powerful than you may anticipate. You might believe that cutting sugar out of your diet is as simple as having the willpower to avoid that cupcake or slice of pie at the next party, but the truth is much more complicated than that. You have likely spent years building up a dependency upon sugar, so when you abruptly try to remove it, your body will react to the sudden loss. Like any addiction, you will start to experience moderate to severe withdrawal symptoms.

During sugar detox, your body protests against the shift in your eating habits. It is used to getting an excess of sugar, and depriving it of sugar very rapidly means that you will experience powerful cravings for its return. You are likely to also experience fluctuations in your energy levels, more common bad moods, and a higher frequency of headaches and stomachaches. Though these symptoms can be intimidating, they are well worth the benefit of no longer being tethered to sugar.

Lack of Energy

Sugar provides you with energy, but it also frequently results in energy crashes. To avoid this, you may have steadily increased the amount of sugar you ate over time so that there was rarely a moment where sugar wasn't providing you with energy. Because of this, you are likely unaware just how dependent you are on sugar for your usual energy levels. If you suddenly cut sugar out of your diet, you will heavily experience those energy crashes that you were minimizing through your sugar cycle.

Low energy is difficult to deal with, and it can seriously harm your motivation to stick to your sugar detox cleanse. When you are tired, you only want to give in to your cravings, and you lose the energy you would need to fight them. You think about how much easier it would be to go back to eating sugar, but you forget all of the reasons why you are committing yourself to ending your relationship with sugar in the first place. If you find yourself experiencing low energy, fuel yourself with more nourishing, healthier sources of energy instead. Choose foods that will keep your motivation high and that give you a long-lasting boost without any of the crash. Replacing sugar with these kinds of foods helps you maintain a balanced state of energy rather than the constantly fluctuating version that sugar provides.

Poor and Fluctuating Moods

As previously discussed, sugar makes us feel happier because it causes our brains to produce more dopamine. When we take away the sugar, we also take away these dopamine spikes. This can result in more frequent bad moods with no easy fix. You may find yourself more easily irritated and more prone to bursts of sadness and frustration. You may also find that you have little patience for minor annoyances that were tolerable before. This can cause you to lash out at others or to turn your negative thoughts inward.

A poor mood is difficult to manage in the moment, but it is only temporary. The longer you go without giving in and appeasing your mood with sugar, the more you will learn to regulate your mood through healthier methods. You may find that engaging in a relaxing activity like reading or watching some television soothes your nerves just as effectively. Alternatively, you might be someone who uses exercise as an outlet for frustrations. Giving yourself a positive outlet for these feelings is very important, not just for your relationship with sugar but also for your relationship with your mental health. Eventually, you will get dopamine spikes from these healthy alternatives instead, and you will no longer be waiting for your next taste of sugar to even out your emotions.

Insomnia

Sugar usually keeps us up at night, and yet, cutting sugar out of your diet can lead to temporary insomnia. This seems counterintuitive at first, but one possible explanation ties back to the energy spikes and crashes that sugar causes. When you give up sugar, you no longer experience the severe crashes that can make you very tired very suddenly. If you once relied on these crashes around bedtime, you may find that you have more difficulty falling asleep, at least for a short while after quitting.

Sooner or later, your body will begin to regulate itself to your usual sleeping patterns without the use of sugar crashes. This process is made easier by waking up at a certain time each day and getting ready for bed at a certain time each night. The longer you stick to this schedule, the more your body will find a rhythm of getting tired at a certain time, and the easier it will be to fall asleep at night to get the rest you need.

Intense Cravings

Cravings are very common when you quit sugar. They are one of the most powerful forces encouraging you to give up on your attempted detox. Cravings may be minor at first, but they can quickly develop into major problems if you don't find something to replace them with. When you crave sugar, swap out the snack for something sugar-free that you can feel good about eating and that you also enjoy. This is a similar idea to smokers who quit by chewing gum every time they get the craving to smoke. You can also minimize cravings by making sugar difficult to access in your house. Having sugar readily available makes it harder to resist the temptation to just open the pantry and grab something. If you need to go all the way to the store to get something sweet, you are more likely to settle for a substitute instead.

Digestive Problems

Sometimes the sugar detox can cause digestive issues. Any big change in your diet can throw your digestive system off, and cutting out sugar is no exception. You may experience an upset stomach or a fluctuating appetite. Either issue can complicate your relationship with food further and make it harder to settle into a sugarless diet.

To minimize digestive issues, you might consider adding more probiotic foods to your diet. Probiotics support healthy gut function and make stomach problems less frequent. Yogurt is a popular choice, but if you prefer you can choose to take probiotic supplements instead. You should also minimize the presence of any foods that worsen your upset stomach in your meals. The specific foods that bother your digestive system may vary, but foods high in saturated fats like fried foods are a common source of upset stomach. Spicy foods can cause similar issues, as can dairy. Once your stomach is feeling more stable, you can start reintroducing these foods back into your diet, but cutting them out for a short time alongside sugar can save you some trouble.

Light-Headedness and Dizziness

A lack of sugar, combined with the resulting lack of immediate energy, can occasionally leave you feeling light-headed and dizzy. When your energy fluctuates and dips, you can feel a bit disoriented. More often than not this is a fleeting feeling that isn't much cause for alarm. If you feel light-headed, rest and wait for the sensation to pass. Lying down can help your body shake the dizzy feeling.

While light-headedness often goes away on its own after a brief period, a prolonged period of dizziness can be cause for concern. If you have diabetes or you are at a risk of developing diabetes, dizziness can be a symptom of low blood sugar. The light-headedness occurs because your body does not have enough sugar in your bloodstream to maintain proper brain function. In these cases, you may need to consume a bit of sugar until you are feeling better, though be sure to limit your sugar intake to a healthy amount.

A GRADUAL ADDICTION

When dealing with sugar, it is important to note that it isn't the type of addiction that occurs after just one taste. It can take years of consuming excess amounts of sugar before you are really addicted to it. Because of how gradually the addiction develops, it can sneak up on you, and learning the full extent of the damage sugar has done is quite a shock. You might not even realize there is a problem until you try to lower your sugar intake, at which point it becomes apparent just how thoroughly dependent on sugar you have become without even noticing it.

Sugar's ability to lurk silently in many things you eat each day only contributes to how difficult sugar addictions are to identify. If you don't typically check nutrition information labels, you may be unaware just how much sugar is in a certain snack or meal. Just because something doesn't taste very sweet doesn't mean there is no sugar to be found in it. Neglecting to read the ingredient list can leave you unaware of sugar's presence in a variety of foods. Sauces are an especially heinous culprit of this crime, as they tend to contain very high amounts of sugar while still being savory rather than sweet. This tricks your taste buds while still flooding your system with sugar. Another example that is particularly detrimental is salad dressing. While not every dressing has a high sugar content, many of them do. If you don't read the label, you could believe you are making yourself a healthy lunch when in reality you are just pouring sugar on top of your salad. A greater awareness of sugar hiding in plain sight can make it easier to avoid unnecessary sugars and choose healthier options.

Once you start thinking of sugar as an addiction, you will find yourself looking back on past behaviors in a whole new light. If you're an emotional eater, you may not consider the damage of what you are doing until long after it has been done. You might hardly notice you've opened a package of cookies until you are nearly finished with them, at which point guilt is often quick to follow. When you make an effort to become more aware of your sugar consumption, you become better at spotting potential emotional triggers for eating. You can then regain control over them before they can negatively impact your health.

Taking Back Control of Your Diet

Decreasing your sugar intake is all about having a better sense of control over what you are eating. While beating a sugar addiction isn't easy, the sense of self-discipline and fulfillment you will gain from the process is worth every headache and craving you experience in the process. The improvements in your health are immediately noticeable, and you will save yourself from many future health conditions just by altering your diet. Additionally, you will feel a sense of accomplishment in seeing just how strong your desire and willpower really is.

People who successfully complete a sugar detox feel great about themselves and their choices. They know they have made a positive change in their eating habits that will benefit them from years to come. Many people who complete this process never go back to their old eating habits because they have learned the skills to control what they eat and have discovered many healthy alternatives to sugary foods. The following chapters will provide you with the tools and knowledge you need to make this change for yourself. They will guide you through every step of the process so that you can experience your own sugar detox cleanse success story and never look back.

2

SUGAR DETOX CLEANSE STEP 1

IDENTIFY YOUR FOOD TRIGGERS

The sugar detox is not a slow, gradual reduction of the number of carbs you eat. When you ease yourself into the process, you leave yourself open to many opportunities for slip-ups. It is easier to reach for a candy bar because you've decided that some sugar is okay. It is also easy to not realize just how much sugar you are consuming if you only take small steps to get rid of it very slowly. You can find yourself eating far more than you intended because those sources of temptation are all around you. Additionally, it takes much longer to see or feel the effects of removing sugar from your life. If you go a few days and nothing seems different, you may get discouraged and inhibit your progress, getting stuck in this process for months instead of the week or two you had initially planned. Worse, you may lack the motivation to continue and find that your cravings are too strong because you are still frequently satisfying them. This can make you give up on the diet altogether.

You want to avoid giving yourself opportunities to

sneak sugar into your diet. This is why the cold turkey approach of the sugar detox cleanse is the best way to start shifting your dietary habits in a way that will produce long-lasting change. The first step is to get rid of the foods you know you shouldn't be eating. If you rid your cabinets, pantry, and refrigerator of all the foods that will tempt you into ending your sugar fast, it is much harder for you to cheat on your diet, and you will increase the likelihood of success.

While it is a good idea to get rid of all sugary foods, take special care to remove your most common food triggers. If you have a weakness for soda, make sure there is none in the house when you start your detox. Don't trust that you will be able to limit yourself to just one occasionally; more often than not, when you have gone a few days without sugar, the allure of a can of soda is stronger than you anticipated. You want to stay strong during this first week of detoxing. If you show yourself that you can make it through a week without sugar, it will be easier to stick to a low sugar diet in the future. Set yourself up to succeed by throwing out the things in your cabinet that will interfere with a sugar-free lifestyle.

FOODS TO ELIMINATE DURING DETOX

The list of foods that contain high amounts of sugars, especially added sugars, is very long. You may be surprised to see some items on the list, as their sugar content is well hidden under many other flavors. Oftentimes you do not think of these high-sugar items as "sweet," but they can interfere with your progress, nonetheless.

Work your way through all the food in your house with this list in hand. Remove anything that appears on the list, as well as anything else that contains high amounts of sugar. It may be sad to feel like you are wasting these items, but what you lose in wasted purchases you more than make up for in the benefits of living a healthier lifestyle free from the shackles of sugar. You will not regret cleaning your pantry and fridge of these foods that pose a threat to your well-being. You will be glad you did it when you start to see the results that come from cutting out sugar. Eliminating these foods from your household early on means they will not tempt you later down the line when cravings start hitting the hardest.

Desserts

In a sugar detox, all kinds of sweet and savory desserts have to go. Anything that includes chocolate, specifically milk chocolate, already has a high amount of added sugar and should be disposed of. Chocolate can cause powerful cravings, so it is especially important that it is not around to tempt you. This means eliminating all chocolate treats and candies. You should also rid yourself of any cookies, cakes, cupcakes, and baked goods in your house. Ice cream is equally sugary, as is frosting. These desserts don't do you any favors, and their overly sweet taste worsens sugar addiction.

Don't be fooled by desserts that seem to taste less sweet but are still packed with sugar. Something like pound cake, for example, can at first seem like a healthy replacement for regular cake. It is true that with pound cake there is no sugar-filled icing to worry about, which is one of the worst offenders on a sugar detox. However, there is still plenty of sugar in the refined white flour used to bake the cake, and many pound cakes have a sweet glaze on top. If you take a look at the label, you will see just how deceptively sugary even pound cake can be. This is true for a number of seemingly innocuous desserts, so use a critical eye when evaluating desserts and when in doubt, throw it out.

Prepackaged and Boxed Meals and Snacks

Prepackaged meals are another big offender of high sugar content, though they are a much less obvious source of sugar than desserts. You might not think that the frozen meal you are microwaving could possibly contain that much sugar, but prepackaged meals almost always have added sugar in some form to improve the taste after sitting on a freezer shelf for months. Additionally, these kinds of meals are full of preservatives whether they are expected to stay frozen for a long time or if they are self-stable for months or even years. These preservatives don't do your health any favors either. It is better to learn how to make fresh versions of these kinds of meals where you can control exactly what goes into them.

Another shelf-stable item to worry about are the various boxed snacks available to you at the grocery store. These could be chips, crackers, cookies, or any number of items, but the one unifying trait is that nearly all of these kinds of snacks will have high sugar content. Check the nutrition label of these foods as you take them out of the pantry and note just how many grams of carbohydrates, which your body breaks down into sugar, are in a handful of *Cheez-Its*. Hidden carbs are just as dangerous as more obvious sources of sugar, if not more so. If you are not careful about your eating habits, having a few crackers could have the same sugar impact as eating a whole spoonful of icing.

Despite their marketing as healthier snacks, granola bars are also full of added sugars. Many granola bars include chocolate chips, drizzle, or a chocolate base, especially those marketed towards kids. Others have sugary additives like marshmallows, honey, maple syrup, corn syrup, dried fruit, and many more hidden sources of sugar. It's a good idea to steer clear of granola bars in general, as they tend to use added sugar to balance out the flavor of the oats. If you really want to include them as an easy to eat snack, check both the nutrition information and the ingredients list for how high they are in added sugar. Stick to whole-grain options and ditch anything that prioritizes flavor over health benefits.

Sweetened Beverages

Sweetened beverages are many people's kryptonite. Soda is an especially notable offender, as it is so widely available and many people started drinking it in their early adolescence—building a habit young. Soda is one of the worst things you can keep in the house if you are trying to quit sugar. You may think diet soda would be a good replacement, but it is usually better to quit soda altogether. Diet soda is still not good for you, even if it doesn't have sugar or calories. In fact, because it seems like a healthier choice, you may end up drinking more diet soda than you ever did regular soda, which doesn't do your body any favors.

Of course, soda is not the only beverage that can contain tons of sugar. You would be surprised by just how high in sugar some supposedly healthy beverages actually are. Fruit juices tend to have a great deal of sugar, both naturally and from added sweeteners. Sports drinks and vitamin water also pack a shocking amount of sugar. While it may serve as an energy boost for athletes, it isn't a healthy amount of sugar to be adding into your diet on a regular basis. Many flavored waters are sugar-free, but others are far from it, so don't be fooled by the implication that all of these drinks are safe to consume. The best thing to drink will always be water, but there are still many drinks that do not contain added sugars that you can use to replace these sweet beverages in your diet. Sparkling water is a great substitute.

Refined Carbs

Not all carbohydrates are created equal. While complex carbs are okay to eat on a low-sugar diet, refined carbs, also known as simple carbs, should be avoided. We will talk about complex carbs in more detail in future chapters. For now, it is enough to know that refined carbs have largely been stripped of many of the health benefits that complex carbs provide. They also are almost always packed with added sugar in the baking process, which makes them a danger to your detox.

THE LIST of refined carbs is long and contains many different foods. In general, it includes bready products that are not made with whole grains and anything made using white flour. This includes white bread, pasta, any pastries and cakes, dough, buns, and breakfast items like cereal, pancakes, and waffles. White rice is also a refined carb, as is rice flour made from white rice. If you want to stick to your sugar detox, you should eliminate all of these sources of simple carbs from your kitchen.

Refined carbs are an especially negative influence on your diet because it is hard to recognize them as being unhealthy. When you think of sugar, pasta isn't usually the first thing to come to mind. Despite this, refined carbs can be just as harmful as more obvious sources of sugar when consumed in excess. Consider refined carbs as "processed carbs" and avoid them as you would other unhealthy processed foods. Take care not to allow these refined carbs to slip past your radar when cleaning out your pantry.

Sweet Sauces and Dressings

If you want to have healthier meals, limit the amount of sauces, dressings, and dips you use. The vast majority of sauces and dressings contain sugar to improve the flavor and balance out the acidity of common ingredients like tomatoes and mayonnaise. Ketchup, one of the most common condiments, is loaded with sugar. You may think that you are only using a tiny amount of these sauces so they don't pose an issue, but the sugar content can add up every quickly and stall your progress on the sugar detox.

Despite the risks they pose, not every sauce is as sugary as some of the worst offenders. Dressings that are mostly oil-based, and carb-free sauces that don't have any added sugars, can still be incorporated into your diet. For example, hot sauce and buffalo sauce are almost always low- or no-carb, and they can add a spicy kick to a plain meal. If spice isn't your thing, balsamic dressings, ranch, and yellow or brown mustard all make for great sugar-free options.

Cereal

If you're looking to make yourself a healthy breakfast, leave cereal out of the picture. Most cereals are made with white flour, which means they are refined carbs with little nutritional value. These only add sugar into your diet, which might make you a little more energized in the morning, but which will inevitably lead to a crash later in the day. Many cereals also add sweet ingredients like chocolate, honey, marshmallows, dried fruit, and artificial flavorings that make them especially unhealthy.

Some cereals avoid these pitfalls and manage to provide a good source of healthy carbs without all of the added sugar. These are typically multigrain cereals that are marketed more towards adults rather than the colorful, sugary options meant to attract kids' attention. While they may seem a bit "boring" compared to *Lucky Charms*, whole grain cereals with minimal added ingredients can be a good replacement if you are used to starting your days off with sweeter options. Just be sure to check the label for any unwanted sweeteners.

Flavored Yogurt

Yogurt is almost always held up as a healthy snack, but the truth is that many yogurts are not healthy at all. The flavored yogurts you see advertised on TV or displayed to pull your attention in the store may be more exciting than plain options, but they are also far higher in sugar. Added fruit and flavorings minimize the health benefits you could otherwise receive from yogurt and turn a nutritious snack full of probiotics into spoonfuls of sugar.

Instead of buying pre-made flavored yogurts, cut up a bit of fruit and add some healthy whole grain granola to plain yogurt yourself. This allows you to control how much sugar goes into your snacks while also ensuring that any sugar comes from natural sources rather than artificial ones.

Canned Soup

Canned soup frequently contains surprisingly high amounts of sugar. Sweetness is used as a way to improve the flavor of any shelf-stable product. Additionally, soups commonly use many ingredients that are high in sugar. Those with pasta noodles or rice contain refined carbs, as do soups containing dumplings. On the whole, if you are really in the mood for soup, it is better to make it yourself. Not only will you avoid all these sources of sugar, you will also have a big batch of leftovers you can use for quick and easy meals throughout the week to help your snack habits.

Canned soups are also very high in sodium, which poses health problems of its own. A high sodium diet puts you at a greater risk for having high blood pressure. When your blood pressure is high, you increase your risk for heart disease, heart attacks, and stroke. As many as "1 in 3 Americans will develop high blood pressure in their lifetime," largely as a product of the number of processed foods in the standard diet (Cox, 2013, para. 8). Dropping canned soup from your meal rotation targets two sources of health risks and improves your overall health.

Dried Fruits

Any snack that includes fruit is theoretically better for you than more traditionally unhealthy options like cookies, but not when you consider the sugar content. Fruits often contain far too many sugars to be consumed in large quantities. The sugars occur naturally, yes, but your body metabolizes them in the same way, and eating too much fruit can still be bad for your health. It is best to only have fruit as an occasional snack and to try to choose fruits that are lower in sugars.

Dried fruits are also worse for you than regular fruits because they often contain great quantities of additional sweeteners. Sugar is added to fruits in the drying process to improve flavor, alongside many preservatives to keep them tasting fresh while still being shelf-stable. If you're really in the mood for fruit, skip the added sweetener and just buy a carton of berries or another low-sugar fruit to satisfy your cravings.

Jellies and Jams

Peanut butter and jelly sandwiches may be a childhood staple, but they are not quite as good for you as you may think. Jellies and jams should be avoided for many of the same reasons as dried fruits. They contain fruits that are naturally high in sugar and can pose a risk to your health. This is despite jellies and jams typically being seen as a healthier option than other toast spreads like butter or margarine. Sugar is often added in the preserving process, which only increases the sweetness of these products. Steer clear of these and other fruit preserves to avoid the high amounts of sugar present in just a teaspoon or two of jam or jelly.

Sugar and Sweeteners

If you're on a sugar detox, it is obviously a good idea to avoid adding sugar to anything you make or eat. This includes adding sugar to your morning coffee, sprinkling it over fruit, or using it to sweeten up a dish. You should also avoid brown sugar, as it poses the same health risks as regular white sugar with added molasses.

Many sweeteners have gained popularity recently as healthier alternatives to sugar, but don't be fooled by these claims. While some sweeteners are indeed zero-calorie, zero-sugar healthy options, others are replacements that do nothing to lessen the negative health impacts, and in some cases are worse than just using regular sugar. High fructose corn syrup, for example, is an additive in many different foods, but it is typically considered to be less healthy than sugar. Honey is similarly full of sugars, and while it is certainly better for you than corn syrup, it should also be avoided. Agave, maple syrup, and palm sugar are also ingredients to watch out for.

Alcoholic Beverages

Most alcoholic beverages contain plenty of sugar. Mixed drinks, spiked punch, craft beer, or any beverage where fruit juice and other mixers are added to the sugar content are the main offenders. But most types of alcohol are sugar- and carb-heavy before anything else is even added. Wine is very high in carbs and sugar because it is made with fermented grapes, and grapes themselves have a high sugar content. Beer is brewed from grains like barley and wheat, which makes most beer high in carbohydrates.

If you want to drink without all of the sugar, choose options that are low in calories, carbs, and sugars. Whiskey and brandy tend to have no carbs, as does tequila and unflavored vodka. Just be sure to avoid flavored versions which increase the carb count.

Too much alcohol can also generally harm your body, especially your liver, and like sugar, alcohol can be an unhealthy way to manage your emotions without dealing with the problems that caused the emotions in the first place. Restrict alcoholic beverages to only occasional consumption to avoid both the sugar risks and the other unfortunate side effects of drinking too much alcohol on a routine basis.

THE IMPORTANCE OF READING LABELS

How do you know how much sugar content something has? If you're uncertain and you need to double check, just read the nutrition label. Many people skip over these labels when they're deciding what they want from the grocery store, but they contain plenty of important information that can keep you from cheating on your sugar detox, accidentally or purposefully. Make reading the labels on the food you buy part of your grocery store routine so you can be certain that everything you bring back home with you is sugar detox compliant.

Start with the nutrition facts on the packaging, specifically the carbohydrate count. Food with high carbs typically means that item will be packed with sugar. But weigh that number against the fiber count, and subtract the grams of fiber from the total number of carbs. Your body cannot digest fiber in the same way it can break down both simple and complex sugars, so it does not pose as much of a risk to your blood sugar levels or overall health. But remember that a high fiber count does not make up for any other sugars the product might contain. Something that has 32 grams of carbs, 10 of which are fiber, still has 22 grams of carbs that will affect your body's blood sugar and can contribute to health problems.

Next, take a look at the ingredient list. Keep an eye out for any mention of sugar or other sweeteners like honey and corn syrup. Also look for other words for sugar that hide its presence in the item, such as fructose, glucose, dextrose, maltose, and sucrose. These are all types of sugar in different forms, and though they may not sound like it at first glance, sugar by any other name would taste just as sweet—and be just as damaging to your health.

Not everything you see in the grocery store has a nutrition label readily available. Produce is often unlabeled, even though many fruits are high in sugar. Reading the label is a helpful step, but it is not the be-all-end-all of learning which foods are good for you and which will introduce tons of sugar into your diet. When in doubt, you can use certain websites and apps for nutritional information on unlabeled foods, which we will discuss in more detail later.

What's Left?

After throwing so many things out of your pantry and fridge, you may be wondering what's left for you to eat. It can seem like you've thrown half your kitchen out and you hardly have enough available to make a decent meal. The good news is that despite how many foods contain sugar, there are still plenty of options left for meals that have little to no sugar content. Diet staples like most vegetables, meat and other proteins, and healthy carbs like whole grains, are still on the table and are more than enough to make a delicious meal out of. Eating sugar tends to lock us into the habit of eating the same few foods every week. Mix up the ingredients you use to break that repetitive cycle and make dinner exciting again. You just might expand your food horizons and find dishes you've never tried before that end up becoming your new favorites.

3

STEP 2

MAKE HEALTHY REPLACEMENTS

Now you know what kinds of foods you should get rid of. The next step is to identify and stock up on the foods that assist your sugar detox. While it may seem that a large portion of your typical trip to the grocery store has just been eliminated from your shopping cart, there are still many excellent, low-sugar foods available. If your diet is restricted by food allergies or the decision to eat a certain way—for example, vegan and vegetarian diets—rest assured that there are options in all different areas of the food pyramid that can fit any diet or lifestyle.

It is important to replace foods in your diet with healthy alternatives rather than just cutting them out. When trying to quit any bad and addictive habit, replacing it with a good habit is much easier than just trying to end an existing habit. This is the same reason why people trying to quit smoking will chew gum whenever they get the urge to smoke. Replacement behaviors give your brain and your body something else to occupy them. Without this replacement, you have nothing to think about other than the habit you are trying to quit, and thinking about it for extended periods of time can make you more likely to cave. Instead, you can focus on building a new habit, which keeps you from ruminating on what you aren't allowing yourself to do.

You may find a whole new menu full of breakfast, lunch, and dinner staples you've never tried before, or you may only need to make small adjustments to swap out ingredients that are high in sugar. For sugary foods that you crave frequently, you may want to have a specific replacement you indulge in every time you get the craving for that food. For example, if you typically open a can of soda when you are feeling stressed or tired, replace it with something similar enough to fulfill the urge but different enough that it is a healthy alternative. You might try sugar-free seltzer or a carbonated water like Perrier. If you tend to snack on something crunchy like trail mix, try carrot and celery sticks for all of the crunch with none of the added sugar. These replacements work best when they are foods you enjoy, so find something that tastes good enough that you don't really miss the food you were originally craving.

FOODS YOU CAN STILL EAT

Once you've gotten rid of everything you aren't allowing yourself to have, fill your kitchen and pantry back up with these healthier options. Give yourself plenty to choose from so you can find a replacement meal for all manners of cravings. If you're open to it, now is a great time to try out some new dishes and ingredients that you've never used before. This can help make your eating habits more varied and get you excited about starting a new diet. It's easy to get discouraged by all the things you aren't allowed to eat anymore, so focus instead on all of the new options available to you. You will see just how much variety and novelty you can still have in your diet.

Meat

Protein is incredibly important during a sugar detox. It helps provide a fairly large portion of your energy when simple carbs are removed from the equation, and it is a great center plate item that is naturally free of sugar. All sources and cuts of meat in their natural, unprocessed form make for great meal options during a sugar detox, and you can eat meat as often as you like without raising your sugar levels.

There are plenty of options when it comes to meat. You can go with traditional staples like chicken, pork, and beef. You can include turkey, lamb, and goat. You may even have access to more uncommon choices like bison and venison. Dark and white meat alike are both acceptable options.

The only thing you should watch out for are meats that have been heavily processed and may have had sugar added to them in a sauce or marinade. Pork ribs, for example, often come served with sauce, but even before that they are frequently marinated with sugary ingredients. Other processed meats like bacon, ham, sausage, and salami carry this danger as well, so be wary and check the packaging for nutrition information to be sure that hidden sugars are not sneaking into your diet.

If you are a vegetarian or vegan, meat is off the menu. However, this does not mean there is no way for you to get your protein while still eating a low-sugar diet. There are many sugar-free sources of protein available to you which we will discuss later on.

Seafood

Seafood is another great way to get your protein without needing to worry about sugar. This includes both saltwater and freshwater fish, as well as shellfish. Some people believe there isn't much variety in taste when it comes to fish, but in actuality fish tastes very different depending on the species and the way you prepare it. If you've tried seafood before and it wasn't particularly appealing, try a different type of fish or shellfish and see if that is more to your taste. Sometimes it is only a matter of adding lemon or butter to make seafood one of your new favorites.

There are many types of fish that are commonly available in most areas. Salmon, cod, tuna, herring, and tilapia can be found either frozen or fresh in most stores. Salmon in particular has recently been singled out as a great addition to any diet due to its high Omega-3 content, a fatty acid which supports heart, joint, and brain health. Don't let the "fat" in the name fool you; salmon is a very healthy choice, as are similar fish which are also high in Omega-3. Other fish options to add to your diet include swordfish, catfish, anchovies, flounder, mackerel, halibut, and snapper.

Shellfish is just as good to add to your diet as fish. Grill or pan fry some shrimp, or steam some clams or mussels. Include some crab and lobster in your diet, so long as you don't break the bank. Scallops and oysters make for good choices as well. All of these are foods you can eat completely guilt-free on a sugar detox cleanse.

Most Vegetables

The vast majority of vegetables are very low in sugars and carbs, which means they can be safely consumed on a low sugar diet. Vegetables contain plenty of vitamins and minerals that are important for a balanced diet, so make sure to include plenty of them in your meals and snacks. You can have everything from broccoli to green beans to bell peppers. Leafy greens are a great choice, especially nutrient-dense choices like kale and spinach. Cauliflower and zucchini are especially popular choices for low-sugar and low-carb diets due to their versatility in sugarless replacements for high-carb foods like zucchini spaghetti and cauliflower rice.

If you're someone who had trouble finishing their veggies as a kid and hasn't grown into the habit of eating them as an adult, mixing up the way you prepare your vegetables can make eating them much more palatable. Roasting, pan frying, and grilling can improve the flavor of most vegetables, as can the right sugar-free seasoning or sauce. With the right cooking method, veggies can go from a necessity to a delicious part of every meal.

While most vegetables are fine to eat on a sugar detox, there are a few you should avoid. Root vegetables like potatoes can be a problem if you eat too many. They are packed with carbs, which raises your blood sugar level with minimal health benefits. Eat them sparingly if at all.

Some Fruits

Many fruits are very high in sugar, which automatically puts them on the list of foods to avoid. However, this isn't true for every fruit. In fact, some fruits are actually surprisingly low in sugar and can be consumed in low to moderate amounts. The difference between acceptable and unacceptable fruits lies in their glycemic index.

The glycemic index of a food is a measure of the impact it has on your blood sugar. Some foods raise your blood sugar very quickly, while others raise your blood sugar slower for a longer lasting energy boost. For carb-heavy foods, "Foods low on the glycemic index (GI) scale tend to release glucose slowly and steadily," while "Foods high on the glycemic index release glucose rapidly" (Harvard Health Publishing, 2020, para. 1). High GI foods give you that sharp energy boost and drop off commonly related to sugary foods. Low GI foods, on the other hand, do not have as strong of an effect on your blood sugar or your mood, so they are much safer to eat on a sugar detox diet.

Fruits with a low GI are okay to eat on your diet. These include grapefruit, pears, cherries, peaches, apricots, and kiwis, to name a few. Many kinds of berries like raspberries and blackberries are relatively low in sugar and have a lower GI as well. In general, fruits with a GI below about 50 are safer to consume on a more frequent basis than those with a GI above 50, but the lower the better. Cherries are notably low with an average GI of 22, so they are the best choice if you are looking for a sweet snack that won't set back your progress. Note that other factors can influence the GI of a food. Cooking food tends to raise its GI, and over-ripened fruits have a higher GI than under-ripened fruits of the same kind.

Fruits that have a very high GI can be consumed, but only on a very occasional basis. Don't overload on these kinds of fruits or you will undo all of the hard work you are putting in. Fruits to limit your consumption of or avoid entirely include pineapple, watermelon, and dates. Even if a fruit has a low GI, you should still limit how often it occurs in your diet to avoid raising your blood sugar levels, but occasional pieces of fruit are okay.

Nuts & Seeds

Nuts and seeds are very low in sugar and don't have much impact on your glucose levels. A handful of almonds, cashews, pecans, pine nuts, or sunflower seeds makes for a great snack. Many nuts and seeds are used in cooking, such as sesame seeds and walnuts, and they can be incorporated into a number of different dishes to add extra flavor and texture.

One word of caution when it comes to nuts is that you should avoid most flavored nuts and go for plain or lightly salted instead. Honey roasted nuts may taste a bit better than the regular version, but the addition of honey and other additives means they are high in sugar as well, making them a less healthy choice. Skip trail mix as well, as it often includes dried fruit and pieces of chocolate or other candy that detracts from the healthiness of the snack.

Legumes & Beans

Legumes and beans are another great choice to keep on hand. They may be a bit higher in carbs than other options, but they are also high in fiber and very low in sugar. There are plenty of options to choose from, each of which can be used in a number of different ways. Chickpeas can be cooked on their own or mashed up to make hummus. Black beans make as good a soup as they do a side dish, and they are commonly featured in Mexican cuisine. So are refried beans, which are most commonly made with pinto beans. Other good options include peas, red beans, kidney beans, black eyed peas, lentils, and lima beans.

Whole grains

Many people believe that cutting sugar means cutting all carbs, but this does not have to be the case. It's true that on a sugar detox cleanse you don't want to eat a lot of white bread or white rice because they are made of refined carbs, which makes them high in sugar. However, this does not mean that carbohydrates like rice and bread are completely off the table. Carbs are still very important to your body's functions, even if some are less good for you than others. The key is choosing healthy carbs and cutting unhealthy ones. You just need to make sure you are eating non-refined versions of these foods to avoid the addition of sugar. You can do this by sticking to whole grain options rather than those made with white flour.

Whole grains are made with complex carbohydrates rather than simple carbs. This makes them better options on a sugar detox diet. Similar to low GI fruit, whole grains are less likely to cause a spike in your blood sugar. You can eat bread, rice, some cereals and oatmeals, and some pasta so long as you choose products that are made with whole grains. These grains include whole grain oats, barley, quinoa, amaranth, brown rice, millet, rye, and buckwheat among many others. If you consistently choose carb sources that are full of whole grains and make sure to always check the packaging of any bread or wheat item to confirm its ingredients, you can skip the hidden sugar that is so commonly found in many bread products.

Eggs and Dairy

Eggs and dairy products are a good option for incorporating protein into your diet and for adding some variety to low-sugar meals. Instead of a bowl of cereal for breakfast, eggs are a great way to start your day. Pair this with a glass of milk for a healthy and sugar-free breakfast —though you should be careful of potential added sugars in 1% or fat-free milk. Many dairy products can be used in cooking in surprisingly inventive ways. For example, if you're making a casserole but you want to skip the breadcrumbs or puff pastry that would otherwise result in a sugary dish, you can mix in some cream cheese to give the casserole stability without it having a bready top and bottom. And of course, cheese goes great with everything.

WHEN YOU BUY DAIRY PRODUCTS, make sure you get the unsweetened versions. This means plain yogurt, unsweetened butter, plain cream cheese, and similar options. Dairy may be on the menu, but sugary flavorings, sweetened coffee creamers, and ice cream are not. Make the smart choice and always check how many grams of sugar something contains before adding it to your cart.

You can also use dairy replacements if you are lactose intolerant or if you want to further reduce your sugar intake. Go for unsweetened coconut milk, almond milk, or soy milk for naturally lactose-free and sugar-free options. You can also buy "dairy" products made with these milk replacements such as nut-based cream cheese and yogurt.

ADDING SOME SWEETNESS BACK INTO YOUR DIET

Many sources of sweetness are restricted or banned on a sugar-free diet. You cannot have many sweet treats like candy, cookies, or cake. Foods that use sweeteners such as honey and corn syrup will raise your blood sugar just as quickly as regular sugar, if not more so. Refined carbs aren't particularly sweet, but even they pose a danger to your success in transitioning to a sugarless lifestyle. Even natural sources of sugar like many fruits and some vegetables are off-limits. With so many sugary foods off the table, what do you do when your body is desperate for something sweet?

You have to get rid of many sugary products on a sugar detox, but, contrary to popular belief, you don't have to completely eliminate sweetness from your diet. There are still many ways that you can satisfy your sweet tooth and calm your taste buds. We have already discussed some acceptable natural sources of sugar for your body. These include low-GI fruit which can still taste sweet without the negative impact on your body, and whole grain bread products that provide slow, gradually released energy rather than a rapid spike. However, these are not the only ways you can indulge in something sweet. If you are looking for another option, turn to the low- or no-calorie sweeteners that can alter the taste of foods without negatively impacting your blood sugar.

There are many different kinds of sweeteners that are okay to use on a sugarless diet. One notable zero-calorie sweetener is Stevia, which has become fairly popular and accessible recently as the demand for sugar alternatives has increased. It is made from the leaves of the stevia plant. Stevia provides the same sweetness with a much lower risk of high blood sugar, high calorie intake, or other health troubles related to pure sugar. Another option to consider is xylitol, which is a sugar alcohol derived from plants. As a sugar alcohol, it is very sweet but it does not impact your blood sugar. A teaspoon of xylitol also has far fewer calories than a teaspoon of sugar, which can help to control and limit weight gain when snacking on something sweet or improving the flavor of a meal.

Multiple artificial sweeteners contain no calories, though you should still be cautious about how often you consume them. If you aren't careful you may accidentally develop a dependency on these new sweeteners that only worsens your sugar cravings. In general, all things are best in moderation, even when their effect on your blood sugar level is minimal. Still, they are a better choice than indulging in sugary foods, so you can use them as a back-up plan for when your sugar cravings get too strong to ignore.

If these sugar-free sweeteners are allowed, does that mean that you can be on a sugar detox and still have something like diet soda? The answer to this question is a little more complex than it appears on the surface. In one respect, the sweeteners used to make diet soda don't put you in danger of blood glucose level spikes because your body does not metabolize them in the same way as regular sugar sodas. They are a better alternative than just drinking sugary sodas and juices, though "healthier" does not necessarily mean "healthy."

On the other hand, the chemical sweeteners common

to soda, though FDA approved, have had some controversy surrounding them for potential negative health effects. Multiple studies have linked both diet and regular soda consumption with type 2 diabetes, with one finding "a significant link between diet soda and the development of high blood sugar levels and body fat, two factors of metabolic syndrome" that could indicate the potential for more serious conditions (Johnson, 2018, para. 12). It should be noted that this does not necessarily prove a strong cause and effect relationship between certain artificial sweeteners and the risk of type 2 diabetes, but it does suggest a relationship of some nature between the two factors.

Ultimately, while these drinks aren't actively harmful to your blood glucose level, they don't do you many favors either. They provide no nutritional value, and since they are diuretics, they don't even hydrate you. On top of that, because they are so sweet, your weakness for sugary drinks may simply switch over to a weakness for diet soda, which still leaves you using food to manage emotional distress and cravings rather than finding a healthier alternative and dealing with these issues in a more organic way. So while diet soda and similarly sweetened products aren't completely off-limits, consuming them in excess goes against the spirit of the sugar detox. You want to make healthier choices, not just choices that appear healthier on the surface but ultimately keep you exactly where you started. You can have sweetened foods and drinks on occasion, but try to keep your choices as healthy as possible and keep your consumption of these artificial sweeteners relatively low for the best results.

EAT HEALTHY CARBS

As previously mentioned, there is a difference between healthy carbs and unhealthy carbs. There has been a recent tendency with the rise of low-carb diets like the ketogenic diet and the Atkins diet to label all carbs as the same thing and ban them all from your diet, but such a generalization ignores the varying health impacts of different types of carbs. You are not going to experience the same blood sugar impact from a slice of white bread as you would from a slice of whole wheat bread, nor are fries smothered in ketchup comparable to a side of brown rice. This is because whole grains are a type of complex carbohydrates, while many sugars that make up other sources of carbs are simple carbohydrates.

Complex Vs. Simple Carbohydrates

Some carbohydrates are simple and others are complex. The difference between the two lies in their chemical structure. All carbohydrates are made up of sugars, but the length and type of those sugars differs. Simple carbohydrates are relatively small structures made up of just a few sugar molecules. Complex carbohydrates are, as the name suggests, long chains of sugar molecules with a more complex structure. The variance in carbohydrate length makes simple carbs easy for your body to digest rapidly, while complex carbs require a bit more work.

The small size of simple carbohydrates means they can be broken down by your body for energy very quickly. If you have a candy bar or a soda, your body experiences the energy boost nearly instantly because it works to break the simple carbs down into their individual sugars incredibly quickly. This is what leads to a "sugar rush" where you feel re-energized and hyped up by eating sugar, but it can also lead to a heavy crash, as your body exhausts its energy supply very quickly. Because the sugar chain was broken down so quickly, your body burns through the energy it gets from the sugars faster than it gets new energy to replace it. You may have noticed that after eating simple carbs such as candy, white bread, or sugary cereal that your energy levels spike and then rapidly decline just as described. Other sources of simple carbs include most desserts, french fries, pasta made with white flour, and white rice.

Carbohydrates that are complex have a much longer chain of sugars making up the molecule, so they take your body more time to digest. You may even feel a bit tired after eating them rather than immediately energized because your body needs to use its own energy to break the complex carbs down into something usable. Because of this, complex carbs provide steady energy rather than an energy spike. They also fuel you for much longer as they are slowly disassembled over time, meaning that new energy is entering your system throughout the longer digestion process. This makes complex carbs a better source of energy for those who have trouble moderating their sugar intake, as you will have a steadier energy flow instead of rapid peaks and valleys. The longer your energy lasts, the less you must eat to stay energized, and the fewer excess calories you will consume as a whole. Additionally, you free yourself from the mood-based dependency that simple carbs can create because you are not getting an immediate boost. This lessens the risk of seeking out sugar every time you are feeling tired or unmotivated.

Look for complex carbs, typically found in whole grain options as well as many vegetables, and try to replace the simple carbs wherever they appear in your diet. This way, you are still supplying your body with the energy it needs without consuming simple sugars that are bad for your health.

Healthy and Unhealthy Carbs

The sugar detox does not aim to eliminate all sources of carbohydrates, nor does it suggest that carbohydrates are inherently a bad thing. Though there has been a recent push to denounce all forms of carbs, the truth is that not all carbs are bad. Some carbs are unhealthy, namely those that fall under the simple and refined carb category, but others do help us get the fuel our bodies need to function efficiently. Without carbs, you would have to drastically increase your consumption of another macronutrient to get the same amount of energy, which could easily turn into overeating. Despite recent popular diets, healthy carbs are crucial for our survival, and they can be a worry-free and guilt-free part of your sugar detox.

4

STEP 3

INCREASE YOUR PROTEIN INTAKE

You've gotten rid of the things you shouldn't be eating and stocked up on the things you should be, but that doesn't mean the planning phase of the sugar detox cleanse is over. If you just cut out sugar and replace it with whatever you feel like eating without regard for adequate nutrition, you may have a hard time staying on the new diet because you are likely to experience sugar withdrawal symptoms. Intense cravings, low energy, and bad moods are all common in mismanaged attempts to remove sugar from your diet. When you are tired, you get irritable, and your sugar cravings return full-force. You need some way to quiet these symptoms, and fast, before they make you give up on your new commitment altogether.

If you're cutting something out of your diet, you want to replace it with something equivalent. When you reduce your sugar, you can also end up reducing your energy if you aren't careful. Most sugary foods only provide a temporary energy boost, true, but if you lose even the brief energy you get from sugary snacks without replenishing your energy in another way, you will find yourself constantly tired and often cranky. Because of this persistent bad mood, you are much more likely to return to sugar, as it gives you a little boost in both mood and energy.

One method for replacing your energy is using complex carbs instead of simple ones as discussed above. While complex carbs are very beneficial, they are not the only nutrient you need, and eating them to the exclusion of other food groups can leave your meal plans lacking, not to mention repetitive. A well-rounded diet is the best approach, so a more optimal strategy involves mixing complex carbs with other food groups that are also low in sugar. This is where protein comes in.

THE BENEFITS OF PROTEIN

Protein is a very important part of a sugar detox. First and foremost, it is a great source of energy. It takes a bit longer for your body to break down protein than it does carbohydrates, so you can be certain you are getting enough long-term energy throughout the day. Sugar withdrawal can make you tired and jittery, but protein works against these symptoms.

Additionally, protein helps your body repair its tissues and construct many important molecules that keep you functioning properly. This is important for everyone, but it is especially important when you are exercising. If you are using a sugar detox to help manage your weight or to get fit, you have likely taken up some form of exercise to improve your results. Exercise is great for our minds and bodies, so even if you aren't actively trying to lose weight, it's still a good idea to get up and move for part of the day. Tissue and cell damage caused by workouts is repaired more easily by our bodies when we eat more protein. This means less soreness, which allows someone to work out harder, for longer, and burn more calories.

Finally, the vast majority of protein sources are very low in sugars. The same is true for simple carbs. Of course, this does not mean these things cannot be added to proteins; a burger on a bun and covered in ketchup is going to have more sugar than a plain burger patty on its own. This just means that you should be careful what you put on your food, and watch out for any marinades and sauces that could be used in the preparing or cooking process. So long as you keep added sugar away from your meals, protein provides an amazing energy source that is both tasty and good for you. It is also one that can help ease the symptoms of sugar withdrawal.

Pushing Back Against Withdrawal Symptoms

We have already discussed some of the most common and most difficult symptoms of sugar withdrawal. These include irritability, energy dips, intense cravings, and a compulsive desire to eat, even when you are not particularly hungry. Protein works to manage and ease many of these symptoms, which can give your detox attempt a higher chance at being a success. The worst thing you can do at this stage, now that you have already put in so much effort into changing your eating habits, is to give up because the cravings got too strong or because your energy was suffering. Eat more protein to control the negative effects that sugar still has over your body during this detox period.

Perhaps the most frequent reason for abandoning an attempt to leave sugar behind is that persistent craving for sugar once you begin a detox. Remember that sugar is addictive, and your body will want to return to it the second anything goes wrong. Cravings for the thing you quit, whether it is food or something else entirely, are very common when trying to manage an addiction. It is the same craving that makes many recovering alcoholics consider having "just one more glass" and causes many recovering gamblers to make "just one more bet." With sugar, you will want "just one more taste." Cravings can keep you shackled to your sugar burden for far longer than you need to be.

Protein helps you quell those sugar cravings, in part because protein reroutes your brain's dopamine production towards healthier triggers. Studies of the relationship between protein and brain chemistry have found that "adding protein to meals helps curb cravings by increasing levels of the brain's reward hormone, dopamine," which in turn "means the brain is quicker to recognise the high-protein meal as a reward, and will remain 'satisfied' with it for longer than a low-protein meal" (Puscas, 2018, para. 3). Your brain rewards you for making the replacement to a healthier food, which lessens the connection you have made between sugar and positive feelings.

Protein also helps limit cravings by keeping you fuller for longer than most other types of foods, even when the protein holds fewer calories. Your body produces many hormones that create the feelings you recognize as hunger or fullness. The hunger hormone called ghrelin will signal that your stomach is empty and in need of food. Rates of ghrelin are highest when you haven't eaten in a while, and production tends to calm down after you eat. At this point, your body produces another hormone called peptide YY, which lowers your appetite. Protein makes you feel more full because it decreases the production of ghrelin and increases the production of peptide YY. You will still feel hungry, of course, but on a high-protein diet your hunger is less likely to be such a powerful force that it causes you to seek out snacks and pile your plate with food. When you add more protein to your diet, you may find your plate size shrinking as your hunger lessens and your cravings subside.

Long Term Energy

Low energy is another hurdle that presents itself after quitting sugar. When your energy is low, you don't feel like doing much of anything other than crawling back into bed and taking a nap. This is more than just a minor annoyance; persistent fatigue can interfere with work, your personal relationships, and your ability to fully enjoy your life. Raising your energy levels will effectively give you more time in the day to do everything you need to do. As you spend less time sleeping, or working so slowly and inefficiently you may as well be sleeping, you will have more time to focus on the task at hand.

Protein is broken down slowly in your body, which means it supplies you with a steadier stream of energy for a longer period of time. Rather than being formed by sugar molecules like in carbohydrates, the building blocks that make up proteins are amino acids. Like complex carbs, proteins contain long chains of these amino acids. But unlike complex carbs, these chains are even longer, are arranged in a more intricate pattern, and have stronger links between the amino acids in the chain. Your body burns more calories during the digestion process of protein than it does when digesting fats and carbs because of how difficult it is to break protein down into its individual amino acids for use. The difficulty of this process means that your body takes a while to extract all the energy it can from foods high in protein, which allows you to receive the energy benefits spread out over a longer period of time. Smaller quantities of food translate into more energy with fewer spikes and dips in your overall energy levels.

STARTING YOUR DAY RIGHT

Breakfast has been referred to as the "most important meal of the day," and in many ways that idea is true. Breakfast jump-starts your day, giving you the energy you need to fully transition from a resting state into an active one. When we start out energized and well-rested, we are more likely to maintain a positive attitude throughout the day and continue to practice healthy habits. These include taking meals on time; a skipped or delayed breakfast can completely throw off your eating schedule for the rest of the day.

What we eat at breakfast is just as important as if we choose to eat or not. A hasty and not particularly healthy breakfast of a few pieces of toast or a bagel fresh out of the toaster might be a time saver, but it doesn't give you the nutrition you need. Even worse is eating dessert foods for breakfast, such as sweet pastries like muffins and donuts. Starting your day off with sugar only makes it more likely that you will continue to crave sugar throughout the day now that you have activated your sweet tooth. You are also much more likely to experience an energy crash in the afternoon, even if you have a filling and healthy lunch. A well-rounded breakfast contains many important nutrients that help us start our mornings off on the right foot. The vitamins and minerals we get from breakfast foods, especially those that are high in protein, fulfill our body's needs from the get-go and set us up for success throughout the rest of the day.

Breakfast is also very important if you are trying to lose weight. When we rest and do not eat for a few hours, our metabolism enters a sort of hibernation mode. If you don't eat in the morning, your body never leaves this state. It continues to preserve the energy you have stored, which means it doesn't start burning calories as efficiently as it otherwise would. This may mean hunger is postponed, but it also means that you're not actually burning many calories during the first half of your day, even if you are exercising. Eating a proper breakfast awakens your metabolism and kick starts your body processes, triggering them to start using new and stored calories.

For all of these reasons and more, you should incorporate protein into breakfast every morning. Ideally, each day should start with at least 35 grams of protein from any source you like. Protein provides a good source of energy. Because that energy takes a while for your body to digest, your metabolism is awakened and kept active, often all the way through to lunch. Protein-rich foods also contain many vitamins and minerals that are critical to our body's function. Whatever your taste buds are, there is a protein source that meets your needs and fits neatly into a healthy, balanced breakfast.

High Protein Breakfast Ideas

If you picture a classic hearty breakfast, you more than likely include eggs somewhere in your mental image. Eggs are a staple of breakfast foods, and for good reason. Eggs are very high in protein and they're a good source of healthy fats, both of which can help satiate hunger later in the day. They are also very easy to make, can be prepared in a variety of ways for every taste, and they don't take very long. In the time it takes to wait for your toast and brew your coffee, you can easily fry up two eggs.

If fried eggs aren't your thing, try hard or soft boiled eggs instead. These are a great option because you can prepare them the night before and enjoy them in the morning without any prep work. Scrambled eggs are another option that can be made very quickly. While omelets are typically seen as a more difficult endeavor, they can be perfected relatively easily. They are also very customizable as you can add all sorts of vegetables and cheeses. You may even choose to double up on protein and include some sliced chicken or beef with your egg dish—but you should avoid overly-processed and fatty proteins like bacon and sausage, even if they are common breakfast items. Adding a slice of whole wheat toast can help round out your meal with complex carbs and no additional saturated fat.

If eggs aren't to your liking, you may find dairy products to be more palatable in the morning. A glass of milk or a similar lactose-free replacement goes well with most any breakfast, including a whole grain cereal with no added sugar. Another good option is a sugar-free yogurt, specifically most Greek yogurts. Greek yogurt is more concentrated, which means it contains more protein. Skip the pre-flavored options and make your own flavoring by adding a small amount of a low GI fruit like cherries or strawberries. Cottage cheese is another potential source of protein at breakfast. Feel free to add some chopped up fruit pieces or top your bowl with nuts for some crunch.

For vegans, eggs and dairy are off the menu, but that doesn't mean there's no way to eat a protein-rich meal in the morning. Smoothies and shakes are an amazingly quick breakfast idea that can still have plenty of protein. Use protein-rich ingredients like unsweetened peanut butter and chia seeds, or make use of protein powder. Protein powder can be a useful supplement if you feel like you are having trouble eating enough protein through natural sources. However, be wary that some protein powders contain additional ingredients and sweeteners that can raise the amount of sugar you're putting in your breakfast. Avoid the more extravagantly flavored powders and stick to more basic flavors, and always check the label before buying and using any protein powder. Another vegan- and vegetarian-compliant option for a high-protein breakfast is avocados. Avocados can be spread on whole grain toast, blended into a creamy green smoothie, or simply enjoyed on their own with a pinch of salt. The options for protein at breakfast are endless, so there are plenty of opportunities to make sure you start your day off with a filling and healthy meal.

PROTEIN THROUGHOUT THE DAY

Of course, breakfast shouldn't be the last time you have protein for the rest of the day. There are opportunities to add some protein into every meal, and when you do, you will experience the same craving-reducing and energy-boosting benefits you get from a protein packed breakfast.

The best way to ensure that you are getting enough protein in your diet is to include at least one high quality source of protein in every meal. You can have some lean chicken breast cut up and added to a salad, or you can make yourself a side of quinoa to go with your dinner. Have some hummus as a small snack between meals, or bring a cup of yogurt with you to work. As long as you include some protein in every meal, you are unlikely to feel that your cravings are unsatisfied, and less likely to miss sugar very much at all.

In general, you should try to stick to leaner cuts of meat and other low-fat protein options. Some fat is okay and necessary for the proper functioning of your body's systems, but you don't want to overload yourself. When you do include fat in your diet, it is better to eat monounsaturated and polyunsaturated fats than saturated and trans fats. This means choosing healthy oils, nuts, and fish over fried foods, high fat cuts of red meat, coffee creamer, and various snack foods.

Non-Meat Sources of Protein

We have already discussed some of the meatless options for protein at breakfast. There are many more options you can use to fulfill your protein needs at lunch and dinner. Plants provide a great deal of protein without sugar so long as you go for whole ingredients rather than pre-made and prepared foods. For example, vegan cream cheeses are often fairly high in protein, but they tend to contain added sugars as well. You are better off using naturally vegan and vegetarian foods rather than plant-based versions of animal products to minimize the chances of added sugar in your diet.

Luckily, there are many various protein sources that are readily available to you. Beans are an amazing meatless source of protein, and they can be combined with brown rice or quinoa for a protein-packed simple lunch or dinner. Lentils are another good source of protein, as are chickpeas and tofu. All of these options naturally contain low or no sugar, and they can all be used to make delicious, filling meals for lunch and dinner.

HIGH PROTEIN FOODS

Protein is found in so many different kinds of foods. When looking for high protein foods without sugar, there are some more obvious options such as meat and some less obvious choices like nuts and oats. What you choose to include in your diet is up to your own personal tastes and your dietary restrictions, but there is a way to include a healthy amount of protein in every meal no matter how narrow your food options are. To keep meal times interesting, try to rotate what food you're using to get your protein throughout the day, and make different meals each week. Variety will keep dinnertime fun and interesting rather than repetitive, which increases your chances of successfully sticking to your diet.

Meat and Poultry

When most people think of protein, they probably picture meat first and foremost. Meat is an amazing source of protein that is naturally varied. If you don't want to include too much red meat in your diet, go for chicken instead. If poultry's not your thing, try pork or something more unusual like venison or bison. Turkey is another great option that has the added benefit of being a naturally lean meat. As previously mentioned, the only meat you should avoid completely is overly processed meats that contain high amounts of sugar in the marinating, curing, and flavoring process. This means most hams, ribs, bacon, and similar foods.

When choosing what type of meat to pick up at the grocery store, you should stick to lean cuts more often than fattier cuts. This means choosing chicken and turkey more frequently than you choose burger patties and steaks. You can have these fattier meats in moderation, but it is better for your overall health to make them an occasional indulgence rather than giving them a starring role on your meal plan, even if there is no sugar added either way. You want to make healthy choices in general, not just sugar-free ones.

Fish

If chicken just isn't cutting it for you, turn to fish for a meal with plenty of flavor even without seasoning. Fish are full of protein and healthy fats like Omega-3 fatty acids that keep you feeling fuller for longer. They also provide many important nutrients that your body cannot function without. One of the best fish to start including in your diet is salmon. Salmon has recently been labeled a "superfood" by many people, and this is not without reason. It is full of antioxidants, vitamin B12, and potassium. It is a great protein source that doesn't have the same saturated fat content as red meat. The Omega-3 fatty acids contained in salmon support both your brain and your heart, leading many to call salmon a "brain food" as well. You can't go wrong by adding it to your weekly meals.

If salmon isn't to your taste, or if you'd just like to vary up your fish options, there are many other fish options that have high amounts of protein. Tuna is incredibly high in protein and can be easily turned into a meal for any time of day. Mix it with some low sugar mayonnaise for a quick tuna salad that you can spread on whole wheat bread for a sandwich, or mix tuna salad with lettuce and fresh veggies for a lower carb option. Anchovies, trout, snapper, cod, halibut, and flounders are all high-protein fish that can either be eaten as a center plate item or used to bring more flavor and nutrition to a recipe. Just about any fish is a good choice, so try a few different kinds and see what you like best.

Shrimp

Fish isn't the only seafood that's full of protein. Shellfish, specifically shrimp, are also very high in nutrients. Shrimp contain antioxidants and Omega-3 fatty acids just like salmon. They also have vitamins and minerals including iodine, selenium, vitamin B12, phosphorus, and iron. Alongside all of these great attributes, shrimp is also a very low calorie food that is still fairly filling due to its protein content. You can generally consume shrimp guilt-free without needing to keep careful track of your calories because they are unlikely to lead to a caloric imbalance.

In addition to their health benefits, shrimp are an especially flexible ingredient for meals. You can of course enjoy shrimp on their own with a little bit of butter, lemon, or a low-sugar cocktail sauce. Alternatively, you can use them as an ingredient in a variety of recipes. Shrimp scampi is a great option as long as you use whole wheat pasta. Shrimp also pairs nicely with fruits and vegetables like spinach and tomatoes. Coconut shrimp is another great idea, since shredded coconut is relatively low in sugar. Shrimp can be pan-fried, grilled, or baked—just avoid breading it, as most breadcrumbs are made with refined white flour. Season shrimp with lemon and garlic in most circumstances and you are all set to have an amazing meal.

Wild-caught shrimp is viewed as a bit healthier than farm-raised shrimp due to the potential for higher rates of mercury in the farm-raised option, but the risk of negative effects from mercury is very low unless you are eating shrimp for every single meal each day. Typically, you can eat whichever variety is available without too high of a risk of negative effects.

Eggs

As mentioned previously, eggs are a great way to get some protein into your breakfast. Their ability to be cooked in a variety of ways means you can have eggs fairly frequently without overdoing it. It also means that they are good for more than just breakfast. Hard boiled eggs can become snacks with just a sprinkle of salt, or perhaps a little avocado and some hot sauce if you enjoy spice. They can also be turned into deviled eggs with minimal work, or sliced up and added to a salad. Fried eggs can be incorporated into a brown rice and lentil bowl as a low-sugar alternative to a ramen bowl. Frittatas and quiches are great choices for any time of day. You can even make scrambled egg tacos. When it comes to eggs, your options are practically limitless for this incredibly versatile food.

Nuts

Nuts are a great snack in between meals. They can tide you over between breakfast and lunch if your energy is running low, or get you through to the end of the day at work before dinner. Nuts are very easy to take with you and don't require any prep work or refrigeration, making them a convenient protein option for any time of day.

Nuts can also be included in many recipes. Cashew or peanut chicken works great with a sugar-free peanut or soy sauce. Nuts are a good topping on salads and on different kinds of finger foods. Pine nuts in particular are packed with flavor and healthy fats, and go great with all kinds of dishes. They can add crunch and flavor to a pasta sauce like pesto, which skips the sugar in favor of nuts and herbs.

Oats

Oats are very low in sugar and high in protein. Oatmeal isn't something you think of when you're trying to get a lot of protein, but it can be a great meal on a sugar detox that doesn't take very long to make at all. You can also use oats in other meals like overnight oat jars and a sugar-free granola replacement.

The only thing you should watch out for when eating oats are additives that could make the meal more sugary. Many boxed oatmeals are flavored with cinnamon sugar, artificial fruits, and other unhealthy additions. You are better off getting plain oats and making your own oatmeal, only adding in what you want and keeping the sugar count low.

Cottage Cheese

The primary protein in cottage cheese is called casein. It takes your body a bit longer to digest casein than other proteins, which makes it a better protein source for long lasting energy. It is also better at supporting muscle strength and preventing the breakdown of muscle tissues after exercise. For these reasons, cottage cheese is an incredible protein source for maintaining energy in an active lifestyle.

There have been many recent recommendations by dieticians and nutritionists to eat a few spoonfuls of cottage cheese before bed. This is because of the casein protein. If we don't eat anything before bed, our metabolisms slow nearly to a halt; on the other hand, if you eat something sugary before bed, your body metabolizes it too quickly and you can find it hard to fall asleep. Casein-heavy cottage cheese is the perfect compromise between these two extremes. As your body slowly breaks down the protein throughout the night, your metabolism remains active, which lets you burn fat even while you are fast asleep.

Cottage cheese is commonly enjoyed as a snack on its own just fine, but you can mix it up a bit if you start getting bored of it. Slice up some fruit with a low GI, and sprinkle just a pinch of cinnamon—not cinnamon sugar—on top. Alternatively, you can use it as a dip for low-sugar vegetable slices. If you're not a huge fan of the chunkier texture of cottage cheese, you can blend it for a few seconds to make it creamier and more palatable.

Yogurt and Milk

Yogurt is another dairy product that is high in protein and low in sugar. People who regularly include yogurt in their diet experience, on average, higher energy levels and fewer problems with irregular and upset stomachs. This is because yogurt is also a great source of probiotics. These are good bacteria that live in your gut and keep your digestive system regular. Probiotics also exist in pill and gummy supplement form, but it is much easier and tastier to include some yogurt in your diet. The best kind of yogurt for protein is Greek yogurt. Greek yogurt has a higher concentration of casein compared to whey and provides more protein to your body in general.

Regular milk is a good source of protein as well. Milk contains both casein and whey proteins. It has many other benefits that make it worthy of inclusion in your diet. The calcium in milk keeps your bones strong, which helps you resist injuries and avoid conditions like osteoporosis as you age. Another benefit of milk is its potassium, which supports a healthy blood pressure, and vitamin D, which also aids bone health. If you aren't a huge fan of milk on its own, it is used in many recipes, so there are plenty of opportunities to add dairy protein into your diet.

The only thing to watch out for in regards to milk and other dairy products is how much sugar you are consuming. Lactose is a sugar, albeit a naturally occurring one, and it can influence your blood glucose levels. However, it has a relatively low GI and it is unlikely to cause your blood sugar to spike like candy or desserts would, so you are fine to have milk so long as you do not go overboard.

Quinoa

Quinoa is a plant-based protein powerhouse. It is generally considered to be one of the best sources of protein out of all the grains, and for good reason. Just one cup of cooked quinoa can put a significant dent in your protein goals for the day. It contains all nine necessary amino acids that we must get from food and cannot make ourselves. It's a good idea to add a scoop of quinoa to your daily meals as often as possible.

Quinoa makes an amazing replacement for white rice as a side dish. You get all the benefits of the extra protein with none of the sugar. Add a protein and some veggies for a quinoa bowl, or flavor it with garlic, diced vegetables, and a little butter and enjoy it on its own. You can also use quinoa as a protein in your salad or add it to various soups and stews. As a tip, always rinse quinoa before cooking, and cook quinoa in a low-sugar vegetable or chicken broth instead of just water to give it some extra flavor.

Lentils

Lentils are a type of legume, just like peas and beans. If you're not familiar with lentils, they can be a bit intimidating to cook because they aren't a common ingredient in most American households, but their protein count makes them well worth adding to your diet. They are a great ingredient in soups, go well with salad, and star in dal, a type of Indian stew.

One important note regarding lentils is that they should never be eaten raw. Raw lentils can be toxic and will likely make you sick, but the toxin in them breaks down during the cooking process so you can enjoy them safely.

Beans and Seeds

Beans are one of the most common non-meat sources of protein. They come in many varieties, each with their own unique flavor and uses. Beans are also very high in fiber, which is imperative in a healthy digestive system and helps to reduce their carbohydrate impact.

Seeds are an equally good choice. Chia seeds, sesame

seeds, and sunflower seeds are great additions to your diet. Many people include chia seeds in their smoothies, and lightly toasted sesame seeds are involved in many Asian cuisine dishes. Pumpkin seeds are another good choice. Try roasting them in the oven with a little olive oil and seasoning for an especially tasty and nutritious treat.

Peas

You may not think of peas right away when you look for high-protein foods, but they are actually fairly protein dense. Like other legumes, peas have minimal naturally occurring sugars and plenty of protein. They are also low in sodium, low in calories, and free of cholesterol and fat, making them an all-around healthy food. Peas make a good side dish to any meal. They can also be combined with other diced vegetables, fresh or frozen, and used as ingredients in meals like stews and casseroles.

Edamame

Edamame are a version of soybeans that involves picking them before they have fully ripened. Like any soy product, they provide a good source of protein, as well as a decent amount of vitamin K, antioxidants, and fiber. Some have claimed that edamame can help lower negative LDL cholesterol levels, (Arnarson, 2017, para. 23). Lower cholesterol can potentially decrease the risk of heart disease and other dangerous conditions.

Edamame are typically sold still inside the pods. Despite this, the pods are not edible, so you should remove them from their casing before eating. Some common uses for edamame include salads, stews, soups, noodle dishes, and on their own as a quick and easy snack.

Soybeans

Like their prematurely picked cousins, soybeans are equally high in protein. They also have many of the same benefits, including having an effect on cholesterol levels and being high in antioxidants and fiber. Unlike edamame, soybeans are a little more versatile in terms of what they can be used for when cooking. Soybeans are a common ingredient in plant-based meat and dairy alternatives like soy burgers, soy milk, and soy cheese. Tofu is used in many kinds of dishes as a meat replacement. Contrary to popular thought, tofu isn't reserved just for vegetarians and vegans. Tofu is an excellent way to vary your meals and take a break from potential sources of saturated fats by decreasing your meat consumption.

The only thing you should keep an eye on when consuming soy-based products is any sugars that might have been added to improve the flavor of the food. Remember to check the packaging before putting anything in your cart.

Chickpeas and Hummus

Chickpeas are a common protein source in many vegetarian and vegan diets. They are also a good source of vitamins and minerals including manganese, folate, and iron. Chickpeas are high in fiber and relatively low in calories for the energy they provide. Many people add chickpeas to salads or roast them for a side dish. They are especially common in Greek dishes like falafel.

Of course, chickpeas are perhaps more popularly known and consumed as hummus. Hummus is made with mashed chickpeas and tahini, a paste derived from sesame seeds. If you are buying pre-made hummus at the store, watch out for any flavorings that might increase the sugar content. If you want to avoid this risk, make your own hummus at home and add only what you like and what fits your diet. Instead of chips and crackers, dip vegetables in hummus for a low sugar option.

Broccoli and Brussels Sprouts

You might not think these leafy greens are especially high in protein, but in truth broccoli and Brussels sprouts can be decent protein sources. They are less impressive than center plate items like meat and yogurt, but adding a side of either of these veggies to your meal can raise its overall protein content. On top of that, there are many other reasons to eat both broccoli and Brussels sprouts. Broccoli is especially high in vitamin C, which supports the health of your body tissues. It contains vitamin A and calcium and makes a good alternative to milk in regards to those vitamins. Brussels sprouts are chock-full of various vitamins and minerals, and they're well worth eating. You may have had bad experiences with them as a kid, but just try pan-frying them until they're real crispy. Then use a liberal amount of garlic and you are certain to put your days of hating Brussels sprouts behind you.

KEEP TRACK OF YOUR PROTEIN CONSUMPTION

It's not always easy to make sure you're getting enough protein in your diet. Even with so many options to choose from, there is still a chance that you will overestimate how much protein is in your meals and fall below your protein goals. Failing to eat enough protein commonly leads to irritability, low energy, more intense cravings for sugar, and a higher chance of giving in to those cravings.

Be sure to eat enough protein to avoid these withdrawal symptoms.

You can keep track of your protein consumption in a few different ways. One method is to do it manually with a food journal. With this method, you write out what you eat for each meal and make a note of its nutritional info. You can track calories, protein, carbs, sugars, and anything else you want to keep an eye on like sodium levels and cholesterol. However, you do have to look up and accurately record the nutrition information yourself, which can be a bit of a chore if you're trying to quickly eat and start your next task.

Another option is using websites and apps to help track your eating habits. With these applications, you typically only have to choose the type and amount of food you ate and information about protein, calories, and other nutrition facts will auto populate. These kinds of apps also often let you set goals for certain macronutrients, so you can specify the protein goal you want to hit by the end of the day or for each meal and adjust your meals accordingly. One such app that helps you see the nutritional breakdown of your meals is Cronometer. This app allows you to input your food choices, keep track of how many calories you have burned versus how many you have consumed, and see the breakdown of protein, carbs, and fat that goes into your diet. These can be very helpful tools when trying to limit your sugar and increase your protein, so be sure to make use of all tools available to you.

Enjoying, Not Obsessing

While tracking your meals is a good idea, this is only true as long as you refrain from obsessing over what you are eating. You should practice good nutrition, but not at the risk of your mental health or developing a harmful relationship with food. After all, food is an inherently enjoyable part of your day. It should not become something you dread or spend a large portion of your day stressing over. While you should exhibit some control over what you eat in the sense that you do not want to consume things that are bad for you, rigidly controlling your meals and their contents to the point of obsession is more common in disordered eating than it is in true healthy eating.

If you have a background of disordered eating habits such as anorexia, bulimia, or binging, or you believe you are at a high risk for developing these conditions, you should be wary about how thoroughly you track your macronutrients and calories. Turning eating into a numbers game has the potential to trigger these conditions as it can encourage some people to harm themselves through incredibly restrictive eating habits and feel intense guilt if they miss their mark. Some will also find that tracking protein through these methods is not a good fit for them for other reasons, such as a busy schedule or an inability to remember to enter data. Whatever the reason, the good news is that while apps like Cronometer can be helpful, they are not mandatory to achieve your goal of cutting back on sugar.

It is completely possible to be successful on the sugar detox cleanse without needing to track your protein or constantly critique what and how much you are eating, so there is no need to engage in these strategies if you feel they may be triggers for you. Instead, just focus on eliminating sugary foods and increasing proteins in a more general sense. Do your best to stay healthy both physically and mentally, and don't put one at risk to improve the other. Your whole system, body and mind, needs to be considered when improving your well-being.

Using Pre-made Meal Plans

If you believe Cronometer and similar apps could trigger disordered eating symptoms, or if you are having trouble sticking to tracking your protein, another method you can try is making use of meal plans. Meal plans give you a guiding hand when first starting a diet by showing you the kinds of foods that are acceptable and the kinds that should be avoided. They give you a good idea of the balance you should have between proteins, carbs, and fats in your diet. Pre-made meal plans take away the tendency for obsession that can occur with meal tracking because they provide you with the foods and recipes you need without requiring you to do the math on everything you eat. All of the work is done for you, and you can focus on making amazing food that is good for you. The following chapter contains a meal plan for your first week on the sugar detox which can be a good place to start if you are uncertain how to begin.

As you progress further into the diet, you can decide whether you want to keep using meal plans or if you feel you have gotten a good sense for the eating habits that are expected of you. If you decide the latter, you can slowly transition to making your own meal plans or eating more intuitively while still sticking to a low-sugar, high-protein diet.

5

STEP 4 - WEEK 1

DO MORE THROUGH MEAL PLANNING

When starting a new diet, it is important to take the guesswork out of the equation. You want a strong start, and that means avoiding any slip-ups in the first few days. It is easy to misunderstand the requirements of a diet or to forget which foods aren't allowed to be eaten, especially if the diet is a drastic change from what you are used to. This is very likely true for you if you are starting a sugar detox cleanse, as previously sugar may have seemed to dominate the vast majority of your meals, whether you realized it at the time or not. With a meal plan, the road ahead of you will be clear, your weekly goals will be well defined, and the steps you need to take to reach those goals should be evident.

A week one meal plan helps you accomplish all this and more. By learning the types of ingredients and meals that are acceptable on a low-sugar diet, you can more easily incorporate these kinds of foods into your diet. Even if you don't like every meal, you can choose those you like and find substitutions for those you don't.

Following a meal plan takes some of the hassle and confusion out of starting a diet by telling you exactly what you need to eat every day. It ensures that you are starting off on the right foot and following the trajectory that will allow you to keep practicing good eating habits.

The week one meal plan also gives you guidance on how you should plan your grocery trips in the future. It is a good idea to do some meal planning of your own once you hit the end of week one. Come up with a series of dishes you want to make throughout the week that sound tasty and also fulfill your nutrient needs. List these ingredients on paper or on your phone, and then head to the grocery store and buy only what you need. This process limits unnecessary and impulse purchases at the store which may not be sugar detox compliant and encourages you to make smart choices. If you have an especially busy weekday, meal planning eliminates the time you would otherwise spend trying to come up with what to make for dinner each night and ensures that your meals throughout the week are varied enough to stay interesting and keep you on your diet.

STARTING YOUR DETOX

How do you go about starting a sugar detox? Is it a gradual shift from sugary foods that eventually ends in minimizing sugar in your diet, or is it better to start off by eliminating all problematic foods at once? The sugar detox suggests following the latter format, as this gets you into the right mindset for avoiding sugars more rapidly and reduces the risk of cravings after the first few weeks which might otherwise linger if you allowed yourself higher amounts of sugar.

Start off your first week by doing your best to cut out all forms of carbs, both simple and complex. Obtain your energy primarily from protein, and avoid foods high in sugars and grains. Continue this behavior for the first three days. After this pattern has been established, you can slowly start loosening the restrictions. On day four, some healthy sources of carbs are okay, such as fruit with a low GI that won't impact your blood sugar much. Later in the week, you can reintroduce whole grains and zero-calorie sugar alternatives like Stevia. This ensures you will not run out of energy, but also teaches you that you can indeed survive on low to no sugar in your diet.

CALORIE GUIDELINES

Getting adequate nutrition throughout the week is important, even while you are cutting out certain things from your diet. You should still make sure you are eating enough calories throughout your day to maintain high energy levels and reduce the risk of crashing or caving.

The calories you need are determined by a variety of individual factors, but some general parameters do exist. Assuming moderate physical activity, adult males should try to eat about 2,600 to 3,000 calories a day, while adult females should aim for 1,800 to 2,200 calories. The difference is a result of body composition and nutritional need differentiation between women and men, though these numbers are by no means absolute. The calories children should consume in a day are different based on the child's age. Consult a pediatrician or a nutrition expert for more

WEEK ONE MEAL PLAN

In week one, you want to follow the basic meal plan outline explained herein. The first few days will be low-to-no carb meals, followed by the gradual increase of carbohydrates. By the end of the week, all foods that are acceptable on a sugar detox will become available to you, but it is important to start out relatively strict to lessen the risk of reverting to your old ways.

Day One

On day one, you want to focus on giving yourself enough energy and nutrients throughout the day to support your needs. You are just starting to transition away from sugar, so the cravings should not hit too hard, but the high amounts of protein should help ease any cravings that do occur.

Breakfast - Green Smoothie

Green vegetables are a staple of any low-carb diet, and smoothies are a great way to get all the nutrition you need. Add in some avocado and you have a delicious, creamy smoothie that hardly tastes like the start of a diet at all!

Time: 5 minutes
Serving Size: 1
Nutritional Facts:
Calories: 452
Carbs: 14 g
Sugar: 1 g
Fat: 17 g

Protein: 36 g

Ingredients:

- 1 cup unsweetened almond milk
- ½ cup spinach
- ½ avocado
- ⅓ cup unsweetened vanilla protein powder
- 1 tablespoon sugar-free peanut butter

Directions:

1. Slice open an avocado and remove the pit. Rinse the spinach.

2. Add almond milk, spinach, ½ of the avocado, protein powder, and peanut butter to a blender. Pulse in 30 second increments until smoothie reaches the desired consistency, or for about one to two minutes.

3. If you want a colder smoothie, use frozen avocado slices, or make the smoothie the night before and leave it in the fridge overnight; re-blending in the morning.

Snack - Roasted Chickpeas

THESE ROASTED CHICKPEAS are a great alternative to chips or popcorn. They pack plenty of flavor without any of the added sugar. Eat them on their own or add them to a salad for a tasty crunch.

Time: 45 minutes
Serving Size: 4
Nutritional Facts:
Calories: 62
Carbs: 5 g
Sugar: 1 g
Fat: <1 g
Protein: 7 g

Ingredients:
- 8 oz can of chickpeas
- ½ tbsp olive oil
- ½ tsp garlic powder
- ½ tsp onion powder
- ½ tsp ground cumin
- ½ tsp paprika
- ¼ tsp black pepper

Directions:

1. Preheat the oven to 400°F.

2. Rinse chickpeas and dry well. Grease a baking sheet with cooking spray and arrange chickpeas in a single layer. Bake chickpeas in the oven for 15 minutes.

3. While chickpeas are cooking, add olive oil, garlic powder, onion powder, ground cumin, paprika, and black pepper to a bowl. Stir to combine.

4. Remove chickpeas from the oven and transfer to the bowl, coating them in the olive oil and spice mix. Return the chickpeas to the baking sheet and cook for another 20 minutes, stirring once halfway through. Chickpeas should be crispy once done.

Lunch - Chicken Salad Lettuce Wraps

With bread off the menu, try lettuce wraps instead. They make a great low-carb alternative and cut out the sugar present in most commercial tortilla wraps.

Time: 35 minutes
Serving Size: 2
Nutritional Facts:
Calories: 480
Carbs: 4 g
Sugar: 2 g
Fat: 16 g

Protein: 48 g

Ingredients:
- ½ lb chicken breast
- 6 romaine lettuce leaves, washed and dried
- 1 cup celery, diced
- ½ cup mayonnaise
- 1 tbsp olive oil
- 1 tsp spicy brown mustard
- ½ teaspoon black pepper
- ½ teaspoon salt

Directions:

1. Preheat the oven to 400°F.

2. Add chicken breasts to a large bowl with olive oil, salt, and pepper. Mix to coat and transfer to a lined baking sheet.

3. Roast chicken in the oven for 20-25 minutes. Make sure the interior of the chicken is no longer pink when done.

4. Remove chicken from the oven and let cool. Dice the chicken into ½-inch cubes.

5. Transfer chicken to a bowl. Add celery, mayonnaise, and spicy brown mustard. Mix well.

6. Spoon the chicken mixture into the lettuce leaves and serve.

Snack - Hard Boiled Eggs

Hard boiled eggs can be used in a number of ways. You can use them to make deviled eggs, slice them up to top a salad, or just eat them whole with a little salt. Knowing how to make hard boiled eggs ensures you have a relatively quick snack you can make with minimal ingredients.

Time: 25 minutes

Serving Size: 4
Nutritional Facts:
Calories: 162
Carbs: <1 g
Sugar: <1 g
Fat: 9 g
Protein: 13 g
Ingredients:
- 8 eggs
- 1 tsp salt

Directions:

1. Place eggs in the bottom of a saucepot. Make sure eggs fit comfortably without overlap.

2. Fill the saucepot with cold water about one or two inches above the eggs. Add salt to the water.

3. Put the pot on the stove and bring to a boil over high heat, uncovered.

4. When the water starts to boil, shut off the heat and cover the pot. Do not remove the pot from the burner. Let eggs sit for 10-12 minutes depending on how firm you want the yolks to be, with a longer cooking time yielding firmer yolks.

5. Transfer eggs to an ice water bath with a slotted spoon. Allow eggs to cool entirely before peeling or storing.

Dinner - Stuffed Peppers

Stuffed peppers are a great way to get picky kids to eat their vegetables, but they taste just as great for adults too. To limit the amount of fat in the recipe, ground turkey is used, but you can use a leaner ground beef if you prefer.

Time: 50 minutes
Serving Size: 4

Protein: 48 g

Ingredients:
- ½ lb chicken breast
- 6 romaine lettuce leaves, washed and dried
- 1 cup celery, diced
- ½ cup mayonnaise
- 1 tbsp olive oil
- 1 tsp spicy brown mustard
- ½ teaspoon black pepper
- ½ teaspoon salt

Directions:

1. Preheat the oven to 400°F.

2. Add chicken breasts to a large bowl with olive oil, salt, and pepper. Mix to coat and transfer to a lined baking sheet.

3. Roast chicken in the oven for 20-25 minutes. Make sure the interior of the chicken is no longer pink when done.

4. Remove chicken from the oven and let cool. Dice the chicken into ½-inch cubes.

5. Transfer chicken to a bowl. Add celery, mayonnaise, and spicy brown mustard. Mix well.

6. Spoon the chicken mixture into the lettuce leaves and serve.

Snack - Hard Boiled Eggs

Hard boiled eggs can be used in a number of ways. You can use them to make deviled eggs, slice them up to top a salad, or just eat them whole with a little salt. Knowing how to make hard boiled eggs ensures you have a relatively quick snack you can make with minimal ingredients.

Time: 25 minutes

Serving Size: 4
Nutritional Facts:
Calories: 162
Carbs: <1 g
Sugar: <1 g
Fat: 9 g
Protein: 13 g
Ingredients:
- 8 eggs
- 1 tsp salt

Directions:

1. Place eggs in the bottom of a saucepot. Make sure eggs fit comfortably without overlap.

2. Fill the saucepot with cold water about one or two inches above the eggs. Add salt to the water.

3. Put the pot on the stove and bring to a boil over high heat, uncovered.

4. When the water starts to boil, shut off the heat and cover the pot. Do not remove the pot from the burner. Let eggs sit for 10-12 minutes depending on how firm you want the yolks to be, with a longer cooking time yielding firmer yolks.

5. Transfer eggs to an ice water bath with a slotted spoon. Allow eggs to cool entirely before peeling or storing.

Dinner - Stuffed Peppers

Stuffed peppers are a great way to get picky kids to eat their vegetables, but they taste just as great for adults too. To limit the amount of fat in the recipe, ground turkey is used, but you can use a leaner ground beef if you prefer.

Time: 50 minutes
Serving Size: 4

Nutritional Facts:
Calories: 470
Carbs: 13 g
Sugar: 4 g
Fat: 20 g
Protein: 36 g

Ingredients:
- 1 lb ground turkey
- 4 bell peppers
- 1 tomato, diced
- ½ onion, diced
- ½ cup black beans
- ½ cup shredded cheddar cheese
- 1 tbsp hot sauce

Directions:

1. Preheat the oven to 400°F.

2. In a skillet on the stove, brown the ground turkey until thoroughly cooked. Add diced onions and cook for an additional five minutes.

3. To the meat mixture, add diced tomatoes, black beans, and cheese. Drizzle on hot sauce and stir.

4. Wash the peppers and cut a circle around the stem to remove the seeds. Cut the peppers lengthwise so each one makes two boats. Scrape any remaining seeds out of the halves.

5. Lay peppers out on a greased baking sheet. Fill with ground turkey mixture and top with any remaining cheese. Transfer peppers to the oven and back for 35-40 minutes, or until peppers are tender and lightly charred on the outside.

Day Two

Day two should follow the same pattern that Day One

started. Keep sugar and carbs to a minimum, and continue to resist the pull of sugar.

Breakfast - Egg Stuffed Avocados

Avocados are an amazing source of healthy fats and protein. They also pair very nicely with eggs. If spice isn't your thing, feel free to leave the hot sauce out and replace it with an extra pinch of salt.

Time: 20 minutes

Serving Size: 1

Nutritional Facts:

Calories: 526

Carbs: 16 g

Sugar: 3 g

Fat: 32 g

Protein: 34 g

Ingredients:

- 2 eggs
- 1 avocado
- ¼ cup cottage cheese
- ½ tsp salt
- ½ tsp black pepper
- ½ tsp hot sauce

Directions:

1. Preheat the oven to 400°F.

2. Slice the avocado in half and remove the pit. Crack one egg into the divot left by the pit in each avocado half. Top each with half of the cottage cheese.

3. Put avocado halves on a baking sheet and bake for 15 minutes. Remove from the oven, top with salt, pepper, and a drizzle of hot sauce, and serve.

Snack - Cold Cut Roll-Ups

Cold cut roll-ups are pure protein. You can use this

recipe as a guideline and substitute any deli meats you like, provided you stay away from over-processed and sweetened cuts.

Time: 5 minutes
Serving Size: 1
Nutritional Facts:
Calories: 390
Carbs: 4 g
Sugar: 2 g
Fat: 13 g
Protein: 29 g
Ingredients:
- ¼ lb turkey, sliced thin
- ⅛ lb cheddar cheese, sliced thin
- 3 romaine lettuce leaves, halved

Directions:

1. Lay out turkey slices to make the base of the deli roll-up.

2. Add slices of cheddar cheese and lettuce leaves to each turkey slice. Roll into tube shapes and enjoy.

Lunch - Lime Grilled Chicken Salad

USING citrus fruits like lemon and lime let you add flavor to a meal without drastically raising its sugar content. Lime pairs well with chicken breast, so try it out in this lime chicken salad.

Time: 20 minutes
Serving Size: 2
Nutritional Facts:
Calories: 491
Carbs: 5 g

Sugar: 1 g
Fat: 13 g
Protein: 76 g

Ingredients:
- 1 lb chicken breasts
- 1 lime
- ½ avocado, sliced and pitted
- 2 cups romaine lettuce
- ¼ cup cherry tomatoes

Directions:

1. Preheat the grill to medium heat. Grill chicken breasts for about 10 minutes depending on their thickness, flipping halfway through.

2. Wait for the chicken to cool, then slice into bite-size strips.

3. Wash and chop lettuce. Top with sliced chicken, avocado, and diced cherry tomatoes. Squeeze lime juice over top and serve.

Snack - Chia Seed Pudding

Chia seed pudding is an incredibly easy snack with very few ingredients required. It's great to make in bulk and store in the fridge for an entire weeks' worth of snacks.

Time: 5 minutes, refrigerate overnight
Serving Size: 4
Nutritional Facts:
Calories: 131
Carbs: 11 g
Sugar: 6 g
Fat: 7 g
Protein: 12 g
Ingredients:

- 2 cups unsweetened almond milk
- 8 tbsp chia seeds
- 2 tsp Stevia

Directions:

1. Take four mason jars or other resealable containers and fill each with ½ cup almond milk. Mix 2 tablespoons of chia seeds and ½ teaspoon of Stevia into each jar.

2. Seal the jars and allow them to chill for at least two hours, preferably overnight.

Dinner - Stir-Fry with Zucchini and Shrimp

This version of stir-fry doesn't contain a rice base but instead uses zucchini. Later on in the sugar detox diet when healthy carbs are reintroduced, you can repurpose this recipe with brown rice.

Time: 20 minutes
Serving Size: 4
Nutritional Facts:
Calories: 203
Carbs: 3 g
Sugar: 1 g
Fat: 9 g
Protein: 26 g

Ingredients:
- 1 lb shrimp, peeled and deveined
- 1 medium zucchini
- 2 tbsp olive oil
- 2 tbsp garlic, minced
- 1 tbsp ginger
- 1 tsp sesame oil
- 1 tsp sugar-free soy sauce

Directions:

1. Wash and slice zucchini into ¼-inch slices.

2. Heat oil in a skillet over medium-high heat. Add shrimp and cook until pink, about two minutes on each side. Remove shrimp from the skillet and set aside.

3. Add zucchini to the skillet and cook until tender, about five minutes. Drain excess water.

4. Return shrimp to the skillet and add garlic, ginger, sesame oil, and soy sauce. Sauté for another five minutes, stirring frequently, and serve.

Day Three

There is a good chance your cravings will be especially tricky to manage as you enter day three. You may be tempted to return to your old eating habits, but stay strong! Add some extra protein into your meals and push back against cravings.

Breakfast - Simple Scrambled Eggs

Scrambled eggs are a quick and easy choice for breakfast that give you a great protein start to your day. If you want to add some extra protein to this recipe, cut up and mix in some leftover chicken.

Time: 10 minutes
Serving Size: 1
Nutritional Facts:
Calories: 418
Carbs: 4 g
Sugar: 2 g
Fat: 12 g
Protein: 44 g
Ingredients:
- 2 eggs
- 1 cup plain yogurt
- ¼ cup shredded cheddar cheese
- ½ tbsp butter

- ½ tsp salt
- ¼ tsp black pepper

Directions:

1. Crack eggs into a bowl and break yolks with a fork. Add yogurt and beat until frothy.

2. Heat a pan on the stove over medium heat and melt butter. Add egg mixture and stir periodically as eggs firm. Cook for five minutes, and add the shredded cheese when eggs are no longer runny. Sprinkle eggs with salt and pepper.

3. Transfer to a plate and serve.

Snack - Black Bean Salad

Black bean salad is a snack option that is both filling enough to keep your energy up in the morning, and also light enough to make for the perfect snack. Mix it up early in the morning and store it in the fridge until lunchtime.

Time: 10 minutes
Serving Size: 2
Nutritional Facts:
Calories: 221
Carbs: 28 g
Sugar: 2 g
Fat: 1 g
Protein: 13 g

Ingredients:
- 1 16 oz can of black beans
- ½ bell pepper
- ½ cup romaine lettuce
- ½ cup cherry tomatoes
- ¼ cup shredded carrot
- 2 tbsp sugar-free vinaigrette (optional)

Directions:

1. Empty the can of black beans into a small pot on the stove. Cook on medium heat, stirring occasionally, until beans are tender, about five minutes. Allow beans to cool before proceeding.

2. Chop bell pepper, lettuce, and cherry tomatoes into bite-size pieces. Mix with beans and shredded carrot. Top with vinaigrette and serve or store.

Lunch - Salmon Fillet

With the health benefits of salmon, it is a no-brainer food item for a low-carb lunch option. Its bold flavors ensure little work is needed to make this fish stand out.

Time: 30 minutes
Serving Size: 2
Nutritional Facts:
Calories: 460
Carbs: 2 g
Sugar: <1 g
Fat: 28 g
Protein: 48 g

Ingredients:
- 1 lb salmon
- 1 lemon
- 2 tbsp butter
- 1 tbsp garlic, minced
- ½ tsp salt
- ½ tsp black pepper

Directions:

1. Preheat the oven to 350°F.

2. Line a baking sheet with aluminum foil. Cut a lemon into thin slices and lay them out, then place the

salmon fillet on the slices. Top with melted butter, garlic, salt, and pepper.

3. Fold the foil so it creates a sealed pocket and bake in the oven for 25 minutes. Salmon should be flaky when done.

Snack - Turmeric Cashews

Turmeric is a great spice that is both tasty and good for you. It promotes good digestive health and reduces the risk of heartburn, so adding it to roasted cashews is a surefire hit.

Time: 25 minutes
Serving Size: 2
Nutritional Facts:
Calories: 130
Carbs: 5 g
Sugar: 1 g
Fat: 7 g
Protein: 8 g

Ingredients:
- 2 cups raw cashews
- 1 tbsp chia seeds
- 1 tbsp olive oil
- 1 tsp ground turmeric
- ½ tsp salt
- ½ tsp garlic powder

Directions:

1. Preheat the oven to 300°F.

2. Add cashew nuts to a bowl along with olive oil, chia seeds, turmeric, salt, and garlic powder. Toss to thoroughly coat the cashews.

3. Spread cashews out on a baking sheet and roast in the oven for 10 minutes. Stir, then return cashews to the

oven for another 10 minutes until crispy and golden brown.

Dinner - Ground Beef and Bean Chili

Chili is typically a wintertime dish, but this chili tastes good enough you'll find excuses to eat it anytime. Unlike commercially sold chili, this homemade option is very low in sugar.

Time: 45 minutes

Serving Size: 4

Nutritional Facts:

Calories: 316

Carbs: 34 g

Sugar: 2 g

Fat: 13 g

Protein: 36 g

Ingredients:
- 1 lb lean ground beef
- 15 oz can of kidney beans
- 4 tomatoes, diced
- ½ onion, diced
- 1 tbsp garlic, minced
- 1 tbsp olive oil
- 2 tsp chili powder
- 2 tsp ground cumin

Directions:

1. In a large pot, add olive oil, beef, onion, chili powder, and cumin. Brown the beef over medium-high heat, stirring frequently.

2. Add in garlic and tomatoes and cook for five minutes. Pour in two cups of water and let simmer until thickened, about ten minutes. Mix in beans and let them heat through before serving.

Day Four

On day four, you can start reintroducing healthy sources of carbs. It's best to start off with natural carb sources. Look for fruits with low sugar levels and low GI. Use these sparingly, but when used well they can really bring some variety to your meals.

Breakfast - Banana Pancakes

You might not be able to have the ingredients that go into standard pancake batter, but with a little creativity you can still enjoy pancakes. With the sweetness from bananas, you won't even miss the maple syrup.

Time: 15 minutes
Serving Size: 4
Nutritional Facts:
Calories: 233
Carbs: 14 g
Sugar: 7 g
Fat: 3 g
Protein: 37 g
Ingredients:
- 2 bananas
- 2 eggs
- 1 tbsp protein powder
- 1 tsp butter
- ¼ tsp cinnamon

Directions:

1. Peel the bananas and add them to a bowl. Mash them with a fork, then crack eggs into the bowl and add the protein powder. Stir until you have a smooth, slightly runny batter.

2. Heat a griddle or a pan over the stove on medium-high. Grease lightly with butter and let the surface of the pan or griddle get hot before continuing.

3. Pour about two tablespoons of batter into the pan and let it cook for about one to two minutes, waiting until the bottom is relatively firm. Flip with a spatula and let cook for another two minutes, then remove the pancake from the pan.

4. Repeat the previous step until all batter has been used up. Top with cinnamon and serve.

Snack - Cottage Cheese with Fruit

Cottage cheese is a perfectly fine snack on its own, but it can be improved with some healthy fruit. This recipe uses cherries as they have the lowest GI, but you can use any low GI fruit you prefer.

Time: 5 minutes
Serving Size: 1
Nutritional Facts:
Calories: 240
Carbs: 13 g
Sugar: 10 g
Fat: 9 g
Protein: 24 g
Ingredients:
- 1 cup cottage cheese
- ½ cup cherries

Directions:

1. Wash the cherries and remove the stems. Cut cherries in half and discard the pits.

2. Add cottage cheese to a bowl and mix in cherry halves.

Lunch - Grilled Basil Chicken

Fresh herbs can really make a difference in recipes. This recipe uses the natural flavor of basil to give the chicken a real punch.

Time: 10 minutes
Serving Size: 2
Nutritional Facts:
Calories: 412
Carbs: 1 g
Sugar: <1 g
Fat: 4 g
Protein: 37 g
Ingredients:
- ½ lb chicken breast, sliced thin
- 2 tbsp fresh basil, chopped
- 1 tbsp olive oil
- ¼ tsp salt
- ¼ tsp black pepper

Directions:

1. Add olive oil to a skillet and set the heat to medium-high. Lay out chicken breasts in a single layer and season with salt and pepper.

2. Cook chicken, flipping periodically until it is no longer pink in the center, about four minutes on each side.

3. Add basil and cook for another minute until flavor is well incorporated into the chicken.

Snack - Garlic Roasted Edamame

Edamame is a great source of protein. It makes for a quick and easy snack that can be easily enjoyed without much hassle.

Time: 15 minutes
Serving Size: 2

Nutritional Facts:
Calories: 198
Carbs: 7 g
Sugar: 3 g
Fat: 6 g
Protein: 12 g

Ingredients:
- 1 cup edamame
- 2 tbsp minced garlic
- 1 tbsp olive oil
- ½ tsp salt

Directions:

1. Bring water to boil in a pot over high heat. Add edamame and cook for five minutes until the beans are tender.

2. Heat olive oil in a skillet over medium heat. Add edamame and garlic and stir to coat. Cook until crispy, about 10 minutes, stirring frequently.

Dinner - Leftovers

You've made it through what is usually the most difficult period of the sugar detox. Give yourself a pat on the back by having leftovers for dinner. It's always a good idea to make extra servings with any recipe, knowing you'll have leftovers as a healthy and quick snack or meal option for later.

Day Five

Now that you've made use of fruit as a carb source, you can begin to include other sources. This primarily means whole grain bread products and brown rice. Adding in healthy carbs greatly expands the number of recipes available to you.

Breakfast - Fried Eggs

You can't go wrong with something simple like fried eggs. This recipe yields slightly runny yolks, but you can adjust the cooking time to your preference.

Time: 10 minutes
Serving Size: 1
Nutritional Facts:
Calories: 216
Carbs: 1 g
Sugar: <1 g
Fat: 15 g
Protein: 24 g
Ingredients:
- 3 eggs
- 1 tsp butter
- ½ tsp salt

Directions:
1. Heat butter in a pan over medium-high heat.
2. Crack eggs in the pan, keeping them separate from each other. When the bottom is firm, about three to four minutes, flip eggs. Cook for about three more minutes, then gently break the yolks and cook for a minute more until yolks are only semi-runny.

Snack - Handful of Almonds

No recipe needed for this snack. Simply take a serving of almonds in a bowl or reusable container and eat them on the go.

Nutritional Facts:
Calories: 115
Carbs: 4 g
Sugar: <1 g
Fat: 10 g
Protein: 6 g

Lunch - Chickpea Salad

Chickpeas prove their versatility once again by being a great addition to any salad. You can customize further by adding veggies of your choosing.

Time: 10 minutes
Serving Size: 1
Nutritional Facts:
Calories: 196
Carbs: 28 g
Sugar: 5 g
Fat: 3 g
Protein: 14 g

Ingredients:
- 8 oz chickpeas
- 2 cups romaine lettuce
- ½ bell pepper
- 1/4 cup shredded carrots

Directions:

1. Drain and rinse chickpeas. Chop up the lettuce and pepper.

2. Combine lettuce, chickpeas, pepper, and carrots in a bowl. Top with your choice of sugar-free dressing.

Snack - Homemade Hummus

Hummus pairs well with so many different veggies and whole grain snacks. Of course, it's also perfectly enjoyable on its own. You can make sure there's no added sugars in your hummus by making your own.

Time: 15 minutes
Serving Size: 6
Nutritional Facts:
Calories: 102
Carbs: 10 g

Sugar: 1 g
Fat: 3 g
Protein: 12 g

Ingredients:
- 15 oz chickpeas
- 1 lemon
- 1/4 cup tahini
- 2 tbsp minced garlic
- 2 tbsp olive oil
- ½ tsp ground cumin
- ½ tsp paprika

Directions:

1. Add tahini to a food processor. Cut and juice the lemon into the food processor, then blend for one minute, stirring halfway through.

2. Add garlic, olive oil, cumin, and paprika and pulse to mix. Slowly add in 1/4 cup of chickpeas at a time and process in 30 second intervals.

3. Thin hummus with water until desired consistency is reached.

Dinner - Simple Garlic Chicken

Sometimes less is more, and that's certainly the case with this garlic chicken!

Time: 15 minutes
Serving Size: 2
Nutritional Facts:
Calories: 396
Carbs: 1 g
Sugar: <1 g
Fat: 6 g
Protein: 56 g
Ingredients:

- ½ lb chicken breast, sliced thin
- 1 tsp butter
- 1 tsp garlic powder
- ½ tsp salt
- ½ tsp black pepper

Directions:

1. Melt butter in a skillet over medium heat.

2. Season chicken with garlic powder, salt, and black pepper. Add to the skillet and let cook for eight minutes, only disturbing to prevent sticking. Flip the chicken and cook for another eight minutes, letting the chicken get lightly crisped on both sides.

Day Six

Keep going strong with your commitment to the sugar detox. You are nearly at the end of the first week! Think about how far you have come and motivate yourself to keep going through all seven days.

Breakfast - Strawberry and Coconut Yogurt Bowl

Adding your own fruit to yogurt is the perfect way to get a source of natural sweetness to start off your morning. This yogurt bowl makes the most of this method for an amazing breakfast.

Time: 5 minutes
Serving Size: 1
Nutritional Facts:
Calories: 352
Carbs: 16 g
Sugar: 8 g
Fat: 11 g
Protein: 26 g
Ingredients:
- 1 cup Greek yogurt

- ¼ cup coconut milk
- 2 strawberries
- 1 tbsp shredded coconut
- 1 tbsp chia seeds

Directions:

1. In a medium bowl, add Greek yogurt and mix with coconut milk.

2. Wash and slice strawberries. Top yogurt with strawberry slices, shredded coconut, and chia seeds.

Snack - Celery and Peanut Butter Sticks

While the traditional "Ants-on-a-log" variant of this recipe uses raisins, we want to cut those out on our sugar detox. Instead, the celery and peanut butter alone still make for a delicious, healthy, and protein-filled snack.

Time: 5 minutes
Serving Size: 1
Nutritional Fact/Info:
Calories: 202
Carbs: 9 g
Sugar: 2 g
Fat: 15 g
Protein: 12 g

Ingredients:

- 4 celery sticks
- 2 tbsp unsweetened peanut butter

Directions:

Lunch - Leftovers

You've made nearly a week's worth of food, which means you probably have a fair number of leftovers already. Make good use of them to save yourself time during lunch.

Snack - Berry Smoothie

Smoothies are just as good as snacks as they are for breakfast. Try this multi-berry smoothie for low GI fruits you can safely incorporate into your diet.

Time: 5 minutes
Serving Size: 1
Nutritional Facts:
Calories: 160
Carbs: 8 g
Sugar: 6 g
Fat: 2 g
Protein: 29 g
Ingredients:
- 1 cup coconut milk
- ½ cup strawberries, frozen
- ½ cup raspberries, frozen
- ¼ cup blueberries, frozen
- ⅓ cup protein powder
- ¼ cup spinach

Directions:

1. Add coconut milk, strawberries, raspberries, blueberries, protein powder, and spinach to a blender.

2. Pulse for 30-60 seconds until desired thickness is reached.

Dinner - Tuscan Shrimp

This shrimp recipe is sure to become a recurring staple of your dinner rotation. Pair it with riced cauliflower, brown rice, or just eat it as it is.

Time: 35 minutes
Serving Size: 2
Nutritional Facts:

Calories: 180
Carbs: 6 g
Sugar: 2 g
Fat: 5 g
Protein: 23 g

Ingredients:
- 2 lb shrimp, peeled and deveined
- 1 cup spinach, chopped
- ½ cup cherry tomatoes, diced
- ½ cup heavy cream
- ½ lemon
- 1 tbsp garlic, minced
- 1 tbsp olive oil

Directions:

1. Add olive oil to a skillet over medium-low heat. Lay shrimp in the pan and cook for about four minutes on each side, until shrimp are pink. Remove shrimp from the skillet and set aside.

2. Sauté garlic for one minute, then add cherry tomatoes and sauté for three minutes until soft. Mix in spinach and cook until spinach is wilted, then add shrimp and heavy cream.

3. Cook for another five minutes. Top with lemon juice and enjoy.

Day Seven

At this point, you can start to reintroduce zero-calorie sweeteners like Stevia into your diet. Keep the amount you use very low, but if you want to sweeten your coffee or have a small sugar-free dessert, that's okay too. Follow the last day of recipes to complete your first week on a sugar detox and finish strong.

Breakfast - Avocado Toast with Cottage Cheese

With whole grain bread, protein-packed avocados, and cottage cheese, this variant of avocado toast is especially tasty and energizing.

Time: 5 minutes
Serving Size: 1
Nutritional Facts:
Calories: 430
Carbs: 37 g
Sugar: 5 g
Fat: 16 g
Protein: 32 g

Ingredients:
- 2 slices whole grain bread
- ½ avocado
- ½ cup cottage cheese
- ½ tsp salt
- ¼ tsp pepper

Directions:
1. Toast bread to your desired preference.
2. While bread is toasting, slice the avocado open and remove the pit. Scoop out ½ of the avocado from its peel and slice.
3. Top the toast with cottage cheese and avocado. Sprinkle with salt and pepper and enjoy.

Snack - Snap Peas and Hummus

Snap peas are easy to eat while still getting work done. Adding hummus as a savory topping gives them a protein boost. This recipe makes use of store-bought hummus, but you can always make your own using the recipe from day five.

Time: 5 minutes
Serving Size: 1

Nutritional Facts:
Calories: 262
Carbs: 24 g
Sugar: 2 g
Fat: 13 g
Protein: 14 g

Ingredients:
- 1 cup snap peas
- ½ cup plain hummus

Directions:

1. Clean snap peas by first rinsing and drying them. Slice the ends off of each pod, then remove the string that runs lengthwise down the pod.

2. Dip snap peas into hummus and enjoy.

Lunch - Tuna Salad Sandwich

Tuna has plenty of protein and great nutrients that are important for your diet. With whole grain bread, this sandwich is a great light lunch option.

Time: 15 minutes
Serving Size: 1
Nutritional Facts:
Calories: 444
Carbs: 28 g
Sugar: 4 g
Fat: 8 g
Protein: 49 g

Ingredients:
- 1 can of tuna
- 2 slices of whole grain bread
- 2 leaves of romaine lettuce
- 2 tbsp mayonnaise
- 1 stalk of celery, diced

- ½ lemon

Directions:

1. Drain tuna and transfer to a bowl. Mix with mayonnaise, celery, and the juice of half a lemon.

2. Layer tuna and lettuce on whole wheat bread, slice the sandwich in half, and enjoy.

Snack - Wheat Crackers and Cheese

If you need a quick snack, you can't go wrong with about five whole wheat crackers and some sliced cheddar cheese. These foods have minimal sugar and they are healthy sources of carbs.

Nutritional Facts:

Calories: 189
Carbs: 5 g
Sugar: 2 g
Fat: 9 g
Protein: 12 g

Dinner - Leftovers

Reward yourself for your diligent efforts by taking a break from cooking and enjoying something you made earlier in the week.

REWARDS FOR COMPLETING WEEK ONE

You've just finished week one of your sugar detox diet! Even if you were dreading dropping sugar at the beginning of the week, you hopefully now see that you can still get the nutrition and energy you need without all of the negative health effects that sugar brings.

Since week one requires you to be so diligent in your restrictions, it is a good idea to reward yourself once you complete it. You don't want to go overboard, of course—

this isn't an excuse to go back to cakes and cookies—but you can have some sugar-free treats made with zero-calorie sweeteners in moderation. Dessert should always be something you limit your consumption of, but it is okay to indulge when celebrating your first steps away from the control that sugar has held over your life for so long.

There are quite a few options for you to indulge in. After week one, it is okay to have up to three glasses of wine per week. You should space your glasses out so as not to introduce too much sugar into your system at once, and you should also avoid things like wine coolers and wine sweetened with other fruit beverages. These kinds of drinks are much higher in sugar than normal wine and will interfere with your goals, but the occasional glass is okay now that you have made it through the tough part.

If you've been craving chocolate, then dark chocolate and desserts made with unsweetened cocoa powder is acceptable. You should still avoid milk chocolate because it is packed with added sugars, but dark chocolate of at least 75% cacao is something sweet that won't ruin your progress. If you're used to milk chocolate, it can taste a little bitter at first, but this won't be a major issue for very long—the chocolate will win out in the end! Yogurt with a low GI fruit and a sprinkle of Stevia is a great option too.

More traditional desserts are still possible on a low-sugar diet so long as you are smart about your ingredients and make the desserts yourself rather than buying pre-made kinds. For example, there are many recipes for low-carb and high-protein cookies, cakes, cheesecakes, and brownies. These recipes typically use a zero-calorie sweetener, cocoa powder instead of milk chocolate, and low-carb alternatives to white flour such as almond flour and coconut flour. Even ice cream is possible if you blend some frozen, low-sugar fruits and yogurt together and chill the results. Be sure to check the ingredients of any recipe for hidden sources of sugar, but if you are vigilant about sugar, you can enjoy many of the desserts you did previously without any of the not-so-sweet consequences.

6

STEP 5

YOU WILL SLIP UP AND THAT'S OKAY

Despite our best intentions, sometimes we make mistakes and fail to live up to our own expectations. This can happen in any scenario, whether things don't quite go as planned at work or we fail to stick to our resolution to make healthier choices. When this happens, it is easy to pile guilt on yourself and turn to self-critical thoughts, but try to steer clear of this temptation. Guilt rarely works as an effective motivator, and more often than not just makes you believe the false idea that you cannot, or you are not strong enough to, change your eating habits. If you tell yourself that you will never change, and that your failure is a product of your "weakness," then you will have trouble recognizing just how strong you really can be. Give yourself the chance, and don't stop trying. The truth is that you are capable of succeeding no matter how many attempts it takes you. So long as you recognize that the sugar detox is hard, and offer yourself forgiveness when you falter, you will succeed.

A flawless sugar detox is very difficult, and maintaining a perfect detox is highly unlikely. You have probably been under sugar's thumb for years, if not decades of your life. To assume that your first attempt to escape it would be a complete success would be rather overconfident. Of course, this does not mean that you should give up and accept that you will be ruled by your desire for sugar forever. Instead, it means that you should accept small, temporary failures as part of the road towards success—to prevent them from becoming permanent failures. Learn to acknowledge your mistake, understand why you made the mistake, take steps to correct the behavior, and try again with your new knowledge and preparations. Your success on the sugar detox is not a matter of "if." It is a matter of "when." Taking a bit more time than you initially envisioned is nothing to be ashamed of. You are doing a difficult thing, but you are doing it for all the right reasons, and when you finally succeed you will feel more powerful for all of your initial struggles.

HOW TO RECOVER FROM A MISSTEP

When you make a misstep on your sugar detox by giving in to your cravings and eating high in sugar, you don't want to punish yourself for the mistake, but you don't want it to continue uncorrected either. Here are some steps you can employ to minimize the risk of future mistakes while still keeping yourself motivated to keep trying to separate yourself from sugar.

Recognize Your Mistake

You can't fix a mistake if you don't acknowledge that it happened. It's tempting to brush off small slip-ups. You may say to yourself, "Yes, I had a piece of candy, but so what? It was only a few grams of sugar and I doubt that it made much of a difference," or, "I didn't realize what I was eating was high in sugar until it was too late. But it wasn't my fault." However, trying to rationalize and excuse the behavior only makes it more likely to reoccur. If you give yourself a free pass this time, what's to say you won't give yourself another one next time? You can hardly hold yourself accountable for your eating choices if you brush every mistake under the rug. First and foremost, accept and own the fact that you ate or drank something you weren't supposed to.

Let the Guilt Go

Once you acknowledge your mistake, feelings of guilt may start to creep up. You may punish yourself for what you did, even if the mistake was relatively minor or unintentional. This is especially common if negative emotions were what drove you towards sugar. The last thing you want to do is make yourself so guilty that the only way you can deal with that feeling is to eat sugar again. If you allow guilty feelings to fester, they will discourage you from giving the sugar detox another shot. You'll think, "I already messed up once, so I'll probably do it again, which means there's no point in trying to stop eating sugar." This is a defeatist attitude that only ensures you really will never be able to make a change. If you avoid feeling guilty and instead think positively about your future attempts, you will give yourself the motivation you need to try again, this time with more commitment to not caving to cravings.

Identify the Trigger

There was a reason why, despite good intentions, you

returned to sugar. What was it? This will be different for everyone and is often affected by the day's circumstances. For example, maybe you had an especially difficult day, or maybe you got a poor night of sleep. Perhaps you had a very specific craving because of a certain location or activity that reminded you of previous times eating a certain sugary food. Figuring out what triggered your intense, irresistible desire for sugar requires a bit of introspection, but only through considering your behaviors and thought process can you ensure the mistake doesn't happen again.

Avoid Making the Same Mistake Again

Now that you know what event or circumstance causes you to reach for sugar, you can ensure you avoid it going forward. The steps you take to avoid the trigger will depend on what your particular trigger is. If a lack of sleep made you more tired than usual, try to make sure you are going to bed and waking up in regular patterns. This kind of change makes it less likely that you will encounter that trigger again. If you had a bad day or encountered something upsetting, see if there are any behaviors other than sugar that you can use to release tension and improve your mood. Maybe this means working out your frustration, or maybe it means watching a TV show you enjoy or hanging out with friends to soothe your emotions. Next time when you encounter the trigger that caused you to eat sugar, you will be able to work around it.

CHOOSE SMALL SUGAR ALLOWANCES OVER FULL BINGES

When you slip up, you may be tempted to just throw in the towel. Since you've already made one mistake for the day, why not get your fill of sugar and just restart everything tomorrow? This mentality can manifest when cravings get really bad. A fair option here is to allow yourself a single piece of candy or something similar. This soothes your craving but leaves you space to think about the repercussions of your action. The danger is that if you resist even the smallest allowance of sugar for so long, when you do finally cave, you may go all-out and binge on sugar.

It is better to have one small slip-up that is quickly course corrected than to stuff yourself with sugar. You will find it easier to get back to your sugar detox if you allow yourself something small in an effort to avoid a much bigger binge. You don't want to cave to every slight craving, of course, but you also don't want cravings to get so bad that you completely derail your progress when they overpower you.

The sugar detox is not just a single week of changes before you go back to your regular eating habits. There is no end point, after which you will be able to keep eating sugar without repercussions. The goal is an entirely new habit that will lead to a healthier life overall. You will need to make some difficult decisions and negotiate your cravings, and that means sometimes doing damage control to avoid sugar binges. You are most likely going to be dealing with tough cravings for a long time, perhaps months and even years into the future. Learn when to hold firm in the face of sugar's temptations and when it is better to make a sort of compromise with your cravings—satisfy them with a small bit of sugar if they promise to let you go back to not craving sugar right after. Building these systems for craving management in the long-term ensures that you never return to the excessive overconsumption of sugar.

FOCUS ON YOUR MOTIVATION

Motivation can mean the difference between success and failure. It is what keeps you going in the most difficult times and what convinces you to try again if you make a mistake. Without a source of motivation, your desire to make any change in your life is minimal. You might start a sugar detox, but your willpower to see it through and to maintain the change will waver very quickly, and you will find yourself right back where you started.

Not every source of motivation is the same. Some will successfully encourage you with positive thoughts of the life you could have if you cut your ties to sugar, while others motivate you through fear of what sugar will do to your body or what others will think of you. It is okay to have a little of each of these types of motivations influencing your decision to quit sugar. After all, the health conditions accelerated by sugar are legitimately dangerous. But in general, positive and internal motivators are far more effective than negative and external ones. Consider what you really want to achieve and, more importantly than that, why you want to achieve it. The reason why you are trying to make a change can be the most powerful motivator of all.

Weight Loss Vs. Long-Term Health

People start diets for all sorts of reasons. Perhaps the most common is the desire to lose weight. This isn't always a bad thing, as excess weight has a negative impact on your health, but it is often a somewhat weaker motivation because it is tied to an external factor rather than an internal one. Think about why you want to lose weight. Is it to make yourself healthy, or is it to improve others' opinions of you? Are you trying to lose weight because you don't want to face ridicule, or perhaps because others have told you that you need to in the past, whether they are doctors or not? These motivators come from the desire to avoid negative outcomes. If you find dissatisfaction in your appearance and want to lose weight because of it, you are likely to remain dissatisfied and self-critical whether you lose weight or not. This can make it hard to stick to a diet, because the outcome that matters most—how you feel about yourself—will not change no matter how little sugar you eat.

If you want a truly powerful motivator, look for one that comes from trying to achieve a positive outcome rather than avoid a negative one. The difference may seem minimal, but when you shoot for a positive outcome, you are working hard because you, personally, want something. You are more driven and focused because the outcome matters more to you. You are working for your own goals, not because of others' opinions or a critical view of yourself. You are actively trying to improve yourself in a way that makes you feel good because you know you are setting yourself up for a longer, happier life. This will give you the motivation you need to commit yourself to the sugar detox.

FORGIVE YOURSELF AND SET YOURSELF UP FOR FUTURE SUCCESS

After you've identified your mistake, you must show yourself forgiveness. You can spend days or weeks getting frustrated with yourself or feeling guilty, or you can move forward with your sugar detox and try again, but you cannot do the latter effectively without forgiving yourself for what went wrong. Detoxing from sugar is going to be hard, and there will be moments where you want to quit entirely. Guilt and criticism only make it more likely that you will decide the effort is not worth the results. You give yourself an incredible advantage by accepting that some mistakes will occur, but you do not have to let them keep you down for long.

After forgiving yourself, move forward with a plan to do better the next day. You can make this process easier on yourself by following a pre-made meal plan, which takes a lot of the guesswork and stress out of trying to find foods that meet your needs each day. Use the meal plan to help you prep your meals in advance if time is something that keeps you from succeeding. If you tend to grab something quick and not so nutritious when you get home from a long day of work, prep your meals on your days off instead so you only have to heat them up throughout the week. Additionally, make sure you are getting adequate nutrition from your weekly meals. If you are left with big calorie deficits every day, chances are your cravings will be much worse as well. Drinking plenty of water helps you stay hydrated and feel full as well, and staying busy can reduce the time you have to daydream about cakes and cookies.

Support and Accountability

Sometimes all you need is a little support from those around you. Feeling like others are invested in your success encourages you to give the sugar detox your full effort. Sharing your plan with family members and friends means you are making an effort to change your habits and they can support that effort—you're not going this alone. There are now others who are expecting you to follow the plan you have laid out and they can hold you accountable for this in a supportive way. It also means they are more likely to accommodate your new diet if you get together for lunch, so there will be sugar-free options available and you will be less likely to cheat the detox.

Having someone else to do the sugar detox with is another amazing way to keep yourself motivated. Check in and see if any of your friends and family members are interested in cutting sugar out of their diets. It is much easier to stick to a new diet if everyone in your household is eating under the same guidelines. You can completely remove unhealthy foods from the house rather than having to keep them around for other family members, and you can share healthy meals that the whole family will enjoy. Having to watch those around you eat restricted foods is tough, and it increases the chances of you deciding you will have "just one bite" of the offending food. Stay strong, approach healthy eating as a group effort, and you will be much more likely to stick to your sugar detox.

7

THE DETOX IS DONE. NOW WHAT?

You have now completed your sugar detox. It was likely difficult to retrain your brain, and you probably had a few stumbling blocks and delays, but you stuck to it and effectively eliminated excess sugars from your diet. What's next? Do you go back to how you ate before, or do you carry on practicing the habits you learned and continue eating with your newfound freedom from sugar in mind?

First, take a moment to think of all the positive results you have made for yourself. After my own sugar detox, I eased my reliance on sugar to cope with emotional struggles. I found healthier ways to deal with the trauma I endured at a young age. I learned skills that helped me start healing from that painful time rather than simply soothing my symptoms with sugar. I was able to focus and address the root of my problem. As a result of this, I lost a great deal of weight by ditching the unhealthy coping habits I had developed over years of practice. I avoided many of the difficult, painful, and scary health conditions that come with excessive weight and excessive sugar consumption. I effectively turned my life around. You have likely noticed the beginnings of similar changes in yourself. In order to receive the full benefits of a life free from sugar addiction, you must continue practicing the healthy eating habits you have learned and never fall back into sugar's trap again.

YOUR NEXT STEPS

The sugar detox includes a more active phase, where you take steps to consciously reduce your sugar and slowly start to reintroduce carbs. After you have completed this step, you only need to continue practicing what you have learned. You cannot go right back to eating sugar, nor is it a good idea to eat foods you know to be unhealthy, even if they aren't strictly prohibited with the looser restrictions you are now following. Continue to make smart, healthy choices and give yourself the greatest advantages you can.

Keep Carb Sources Healthy

It's okay to eat carbs, but make sure you're getting them from whole foods and other natural sources. Not all carbs are good for you. You can eat whole wheat pasta and whole grain bread, but finishing your sugar detox is no excuse to rush to McDonald's to get a burger, fries, and soda.

Sugars that naturally occur in whole grains, vegetables, and some fruits are okay, while less healthy alternatives should be avoided. Remember to check the glycemic index (GI) of any sugary fruit before eating it, and if you do eat something high in sugar, try to limit your consumption. For example, stick to one half rather than having a whole apple. Carbs in general are perfectly fine, but carbs that negatively impact your blood sugar and cause it to spike can send you back into a sugar addiction over time.

Continue to Restrict Added Sugars

Naturally occurring sugars are okay to reintroduce into your diet, even from sources like sweet fruits, but you should still limit or entirely restrict the amount of added sugar you eat. Added sugars directly interfere with any food's health benefits and greatly increase the chance of falling back into sugar addiction. You can avoid them by limiting your consumption of prepackaged food and pre-made meals, instead choosing whole ingredients without sauces and added flavorings.

The one exception to this is zero-calorie sweeteners, which can generally be used without too much risk of triggering your sugar addiction once again. They do not affect your blood sugar levels, so they don't cause your energy or mood to spike quite as dangerously as other sources of sugar. They are okay to consume in moderate amounts, though you should still prioritize whole foods.

Stick to Homemade Meals as Often as Possible

The sugar detox likely made you more familiar with cooking your own meals if you tended to buy pre-made meals previously. This is a good habit to maintain after the detox. When making your own meals, you get to decide exactly what goes into them and what doesn't make the cut. You can leave added sugars out of the picture and only buy ingredients that are well suited for a low sugar lifestyle. The meals you make will be completely free of harmful additives so you can be sure you are serving yourself and your family a healthy meal that you can be proud of.

For busy weeks, make use of meal prep on the weekends, or use a slow cooker to have a meal ready to eat by the time you get home. There are also many quick, simple meals you can make without much time commitment. A sliced protein cooks much faster than a whole chicken breast or steak, and pan-frying is typically quicker than baking. If you throw together a sliced protein, some diced vegetables, and brown rice that you cooked in bulk on the weekends, you can have a healthy and filling stir-fry in as little as 20 minutes. Egg dishes also cook very quickly, as do most seafood options. Cooking for yourself on a tight schedule is not nearly as difficult as it sounds at first.

MONITOR YOUR SWEET TOOTH

It's important to recognize that sugar may continue to be a temptation even after the sugar detox is done. You may not be addicted to sugar any longer, but if you indulge in it too often, you can build up the same habits that led to addiction in the first place and need to go through the detox all over again. Still, over time your cravings for sugar will lessen as you put distance between sugar and yourself. The longer you resist going back to sugar, the easier it will be to continue doing so.

That being said, it is okay to have a little bit of sugar here and there so long as sugar does not control your eating habits. Many people are able to have a healthy relationship with sugar, even after being trapped in a sugar addiction. It's alright to have a few bites of cake at a birthday party or to reward yourself with a sugary drink every once in a while, but try to keep the overall level of sugar you consume to a minimum. Continue checking labels and keeping an eye out for hidden sugars so you don't slip back into old habits without even realizing your sugar consumption is increasing.

You can help limit the amount of sugar you consume by looking for new, exciting recipes every day. There are thousands of low-carb and low-sugar recipes. Trying something new keeps your excitement for food high, even when these foods have next to no sugar in them. The culinary world is immense, filled with uncountable recipes that taste amazing without putting your health in jeopardy. Make use of all recipes available to you and keep your meals varied so you never have to resort to sugar for a quick mood boost ever again.

AFTERWORD

Learning to separate yourself from sugar isn't always an easy choice to make. It is usually one that requires you to confront the reality of just how heavily sugar has impacted your life and your health. If you use sugar as a crutch for dealing with emotional distress, part of the detox process involves looking at the behaviors and situations that trigger sugar cravings and finding ways to deal with these issues. Despite its difficulty, leaving your sugar addiction behind is always worth the effort, and you will experience a much higher quality of life when you are no longer dependent on sugar for happiness.

Throughout this book, you have learned all of the ways sugar can sneak into your diet—and the steps you must take to ensure added sugars are banned from your kitchen. You have seen the importance of alternatives like complex carbohydrates and protein. You have given yourself the tools for sugar detox success on a sugar detox, including a meal plan, positive motivators for your new

AFTERWORD

diet, and the strength to deal with slip-ups. All that is left is for you to put this information into practice.

You are fully capable of cutting sugar and all of its negative health repercussions. It will take some trial and error, and there may be moments when you are tempted to give up on your attempt, but if you keep motivated and try again you will get to enjoy all of the health benefits of a sugar-free lifestyle. Live a healthier, happier life, and move on from your sugar addiction.

If you found this book to be beneficial in your journey to lessen your reliance on sugar, consider giving it a positive review. This helps others benefit from the sugar detox, letting many people learn how to take back control of their diets—just as you have.

REFERENCES

AlexanderStein. (2013, Sept. 19). *Dark chocolate*. Pixabay. https://pixabay.com/photos/chocolate-dark-coffee-confiserie-183543/

Arnarson, A. (2017, Feb. 1). *8 surprising health benefits of edamame*. Healthline. https://www.healthline.com/nutrition/edamame-benefits#section3

ArtCoreStudios. (2016, Dec. 29). *Banana pancakes*. Pixabay. https://pixabay.com/photos/pancakes-banana-breakfast-food-1931089/

Congerdesign. (2014, Dec. 20). *Mixed vegetables*. Pixabay. https://pixabay.com/photos/vegetables-knife-paprika-573961/

Cox, L. (2013, May 30). *Why is too much salt bad for you?* Live Science. https://www.livescience.com/36256-salt-bad-health.html

Difisher. (2018, June 16). *Kitchen pantry*. Pixabay. https://pixabay.com/photos/fridge-fridge-door-refrigerator-3475996/

Djanoff. (2018, July 5). *Roasted chickpeas*. Pixabay.

https://pixabay.com/photos/roasted-chickpeas-healthy-recipes-3516806/

Harrar, S. (2019, Mar. 29). *Insulin resistance causes and symptoms.* EndocrineWeb. https://www.endocrineweb.com/conditions/type-2-diabetes/insulin-resistance-causes-symptoms

Harvard Health Publishing. (2020, Jan. 6). *Glycemic index for 60+ foods.* https://www.health.harvard.edu/diseases-and-conditions/glycemic-index-and-glycemic-load-for-100-foods

Johnson, J. (2018, Sept. 26). *What to know about diet soda and diabetes.* Medical News Today. https://www.medicalnewstoday.com/articles/310909#diet-soda-and-diabetes

Murray, K. (2020, Apr. 29). *Sugar addiction.* Addiction Center. https://www.addictioncenter.com/drugs/sugar-addiction/

Oldmermaid. (2016, Feb. 8). *White flour pasta.* Pixabay. https://pixabay.com/photos/pasta-fettuccine-food-italian-1181189/

Pexels. (2017, Mar. 27). *Healthy carbs.* Pixabay. https://pixabay.com/photos/bread-breakfast-dinner-wholesome-2178874/

PhotoMIX-Company. (2016, May 24). *Strawberry smoothie.* Pixabay. https://pixabay.com/photos/strawberry-drink-kefir-the-drink-1411374/

Puscas, C. (2018, Feb. 13). *9 high-protein foods that will kill your sugar cravings.* Feedr. https://blog.feedr.co/blog/9-high-protein-foods-to-kill-sugar-cravings/

Santos-Longhurst, A. (2018, Nov. 26). *How to beat sugar detox symptoms and feel better than ever.* Healthline. https://www.healthline.com/health/sugar-detox-symptoms

Stevepb. (2016, Aug. 25). *Dairy products*. Pixabay. https://pixabay.com/photos/refrigerator-fridge-cold-storage-1619676/

Wow_Pho. (2016, Apr. 21). *Grilled chicken and salad*. Pixabay. https://pixabay.com/photos/grilled-chicken-quinoa-salad-1334632/

www.ingramcontent.com/pod-product-compliance
Lightning Source LLC
Chambersburg PA
CBHW020521080526
44583CB00013B/685